COUNSELING CONSULTANTS

The Acting-Out Elderly

COUNSELING CONSULTANTS

The *Advanced Models and Practice in Aged Care* series:

Number 1

The Acting-Out Elderly edited by Miriam K. Aronson, Ruth Bennett, and Barry J. Gurland

Number 2

Coordinated Service Delivery Systems for the Elderly: New Approaches for Care & Referral edited by Ruth Bennett and Barry J. Gurland

Number 3

Aging & Communication: Problems in Management edited by Carol N. Wilder and Barbara E. Weinstein

Series Editors: Ruth Bennett, PhD, and Barry J. Gurland, MD

Advanced Models and Practice in Aged Care
Number 1

The Acting-Out Elderly

Edited by

Miriam K. Aronson, EdD
Director, Long Term Care Gerontology Center
Albert Einstein College of Medicine

Ruth Bennett, PhD
Deputy Director, Center for Geriatrics and Gerontology
Columbia University

Barry J. Gurland, MD
Director, Center for Geriatrics and Gerontology
Columbia University

QUEENS UNIVERSITY
OF CHARLOTTE
EVERETT LIBRARY
1900 SELWYN AVE.
CHARLOTTE, NC 28274

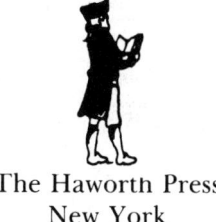

The Haworth Press
New York

Copyright © 1983 by The Haworth Press, Inc. All rights reserved. No part of this work may be reproduced or utilized in any form or by any means, electronic or mechanical, including photocopying, microfilm, and recording, or by any information storage and retrieval system, without permission in writing from the publisher.

The Haworth Press, Inc., 28 East 22 Street, New York, NY 10010

Library of Congress Cataloging in Publication Data
Main entry under title:

The Acting-out elderly.

   (Advanced models and practice in aged care ; no. 1)
   Bibliography: p.
   1. Geriatric psychiatry. 2. Aged—Mental health. 3. Aged—Services for.
4. Acting out (Psychology). I. Aronson, Miriam K. II. Bennett, Ruth, 1939–
III. Gurland, Barry J. IV. Series. [DNLM: 1. Acting out. 2. Aged—Psychology.
3. Mental disorders—In old age. WM 193.5.A2 A188]
RC451.4.A5A3 1982   362.2'0880565   82-23430
ISBN 0-917724-76-3

Printed in the United States of America

CONTENTS

PART I
AN OVERVIEW

The Acting-Out Elderly: An Overview 3
Miriam K. Aronson

PART II
IDENTIFYING THE ACTING-OUT ELDERLY

Prologue 17

How Does the Community Agency Deal
   with the Acting-Out Elderly on a Day-to-Day Basis? 19
Sophie Weiner

Behavior Problems Encountered in Adult Homes 29
Alvin Mesnikoff
David Wilder

Epilogue 39

PART III

SOME FORMS OF ACTING-OUT BEHAVIOR

Prologue	43
The Socially Isolated Elderly 　*Ruth Bennett*	45
Suicide among the Elderly 　*Barry J. Gurland* 　*Peter S. Cross*	55
Epilogue	67

PART IV

THEORETICAL AND PRACTICAL CONSIDERATIONS IN DEALING WITH THE HARD-TO-MANAGE

Prologue	71
Policy and Ethical Concerns Regarding Interventions with the Acting-Out Elderly 　*Monsignor Charles Fahey*	73
Reflections on the Hard-to-Manage Elderly 　*Marcella Bakur Weiner*	79
"Forcing" Services: What Can You Do for the Unwilling Client 　*Rochelle Lipkowitz*	85
Epilogue	97

PART V

A PRAGMATIC APPROACH TO THE MENTALLY FRAIL ELDERLY

Prologue	101
The Case of the Bronx Mobile Geriatric Crisis Team *Sophie Weiner*	103
The Community Support System Programs: A Model for Serving the Mentally Frail in Adult Homes *Alvin Mesnikoff* *David Wilder*	107
The Case of the ICD Day Care Program *Kenneth Pommerenck*	111
Mobilizing the Family *Miriam K. Aronson*	117

PART VI

SUMMARY AND CONCLUSIONS

Summary and Conclusions *Miriam K. Aronson* *Ruth Bennett* *Barry J. Gurland*	125
Bibliography	129

The Acting-Out Elderly

Part I

AN OVERVIEW

The Acting-Out Elderly: An Overview

Miriam K. Aronson, EdD

Who Are the Acting-Out Elderly?

Acting-out is not a singular or even a well-defined entity among the elderly. Rather, it comprises a spectrum of problems in elderly persons who may be described variously as "at-risk," "vulnerable," "frail," "impaired," "disabled," "antisocial," and "hard-to-manage." These are persons with multiple problems—physical, psychological, economic, social, environmental, and familial. These problems are generally overlapping and interrelated; they are incapacitated by a combination of physical and other problems. They are not necessarily discharged mental patients who have multiple problems. Some may have previous psychiatric histories; some may not. Some may have educational and cultural limitations; some may not. Some may have financial difficulties; others may not. Some may have dementing illness; others may not. Some acting-out elderly may be merely obnoxious; they may be actually quite bizarre. These older persons are often socially disadvantaged, perhaps even socially isolated. While many of these persons may have been loners all their lives, some may have become isolated by their circumstances in later life. Alcohol and/or drug abuse may be part of their constellation of problems. It is not uncommon for them to be at risk for suicide. Assaultive/abusive behavior often occurs, but some are quiet and withdrawn. Their judgment may be impaired, yet they may not be impaired enough to be considered legally incompetent.

Miriam K. Aronson is Director, Long Term Care Gerontology Center, Albert Einstein College of Medicine.

Though their need for services may be apparent to others, they may be resistant to accepting help and hostile to those offering assistance. If they do agree to accept services, they may be difficult to help because of their multifaceted problems. For these reasons, they may receive sporadic fragmented care by multiple agencies or may manage to slip through the cracks and receive no care at all. They may be a source of frustration to helping professionals for many reasons and are, in general, a challenge to the service system.

A Challenge to Professionals' Assumptions

The acting-out elderly challenge several basic assumptions of professionals. It is generally assumed that people will seek help in times of need. These elderly persons, however, may manage to fade into the background just when their need is the greatest. Professionals assume that they will be able to perform some positive interventions, but these clients may not perceive these services as helpful and may, at times, actually run away. Witness the bag lady who "escapes" from the women's shelter after a social worker has spent hours—or even days— arranging the admission. Furthermore, the professional often assumes that a client's milieu will be "improved" by effecting a move, yet the client may not agree with the notion about what is a preferable life-style. Some clients may actually prefer what appears to be a cluttered, disorganized hovel to a "luxurious" health-related facility. Some may even prefer a setting that is physically unacceptable by most standards. Mr. C. is a memorable example:

> Mr. C., age 68, lived in an abandoned building with no electricity or heat. He was brought to the attention of an outreach program whose case worker visited him at home. The case worker was appalled by the lack of basic amenities. A plan was developed to try to get him badly needed medical treatment and expedited placement in public housing. He managed to be away when the case worker came for a return visit to solidify the plans they had discussed and systematically managed

to avoid several subsequent attempts to meet with him again.

Moreover, it is often assumed that because this group is needy, professional intervention is required. This group does indeed have needs which may at times be of an apparent emergency nature. These needs are often quite concrete—housing, food, clothing, money, medical care—and may necessitate pragmatic interventions rather than employment of traditional "therapeutic" modalities. Some professionals may tend to shun these patients because they need "only" these concrete things. Some programs may, in fact, be based on a medical rather than a social model and may not recognize these persons as appropriate clients at all.

> A 90-year-old client of a community mental health center outreach program was found to have no food in her refrigerator when her therapist made a home visit. The therapeutic intervention that day consisted of marketing by the social worker who made the home visit.
>
> Certain programs might not accept this type of client or might terminate her after an initial evaluation.

If the agency does not reject the client, the client may reject the agency. There may be resistance or frank opposition to accepting services on the part of these persons in the face of what appears to be overwhelming, even life-threatening, need.

> A street person comes in the emergency room with a gangrenous limb. When told he will require admission, he decides to leave and return to the street.

The needy person who refuses services is not only a challenge to the medical and social service systems but may become a challenge to the legal system as well. When does autonomy change from a positive attribute to a destructive force? Who is to decide when and if to force services? What would be the most effective intervention? How much can be done within the framework of the present system and how much must be done simultaneously to change it?

Another common assumption is that not being able to "go it alone" may be perceived by the professional as a sign of weakness. The needs of this segment of the elderly are complex and often cross disciplinary lines, requiring a series of interventions by a diverse group of professionals and paraprofessionals from various agencies and services.

Another common assumption is the desirability of development of rapport and regular contacts. While ongoing services may seem appropriate, these persons may accept only sporadic intervention in times of crisis.

The existence of informal supports to help persons survive is another common assumption. For many of these elderly, however, natural support networks may be almost nonexistent. Families may be estranged, difficult to enlist, and even hostile. This estrangement may stem from lifelong deviant behavior or, in some cases, from dramatic changes in response to recent events, such as in the following case history:

> Mr. A. was a 70-year-old retired tailor who had nursed his wife through a long terminal illness. For a while after her death he had apparently functioned quite well; however, he gradually became withdrawn and estranged from his family, friends, and neighbors. Ultimately he became reclusive, and his relationship with his sons deteriorated to the point that his sons merely dropped food in the kitchen of his apartment. He refused to even leave the bedroom to acknowledge their visits. The sons began to worry and eventually contacted a senior citizens mental health program. When a home visit was made, a diminutive, poorly nourished, frightened man with a knee-length beard and similarly long hair peered cautiously out the bedroom door. He had to be approached gently and cautiously coaxed out of the bedroom. The sons had to be counselled and supported regarding initiating psychiatric intervention for their father.

This family eventually managed to seek help; however, estranged families may actually prevent or sabotage any treatment for their impaired older member such as in the following case:

> Mrs. C. was a moderately demented, 75-year-old woman residing in an apartment, where, due to clutter, she essentially lived on a couch in the entry hall. She had a part-time homemaker and was receiving some meals on wheels from a neighborhood agency as well. A home visit by a mental health outreach team for assessment of her apparently impaired health was requested by the meals on wheels agency. Her legs were seriously infected to the point of having maggots, and immediate medical treatment was advised. She refused to consent to treatment. The only remaining kin, a niece, not only refused to attempt to enlist her aunt's cooperation in obtaining treatment but also was suspicious of the outreach team and requested that it refrain from providing any services until she called back —which she never did.

Sometimes the families may be responding to their feelings of fear or frustration; other times they may be expressing anger or ambivalence. In a certain small percentage of the cases, there may be financial considerations which may result in inaction.

Just a families may be estranged, so too may peers, neighbors, and friends be turned off. Many older persons tend to try to hold on to their youth by identifying with younger and more healthy persons and thus often hold strong negative stereotypes about aging (Bultena and Powers, 1979). Consequently, they are quite rejecting of their less attractive, less fortunate peers.

Oftentimes the professional may experience fear or frustration. These are not easy people to deal with. Their problems are complex and often defy solution. As professionals, we have a mandate to help, and in some of these situations, we may find ourselves feeling utterly helpless. For example, suicide is a particularly difficult problem for helping professionals at all levels, and this is a population that is at risk for suicide. There is invariably difficulty in assessing the severity of the potential risk. Once an assessment is made, there is often what is perceived as inappropriate medical backup or no backup at all. The emotionality of suicide threats sometimes makes it hard for the line worker to accept the decisions of supervising staff. Indeed clients' fear and pain are often shared by the professionals who try to serve them. As Dr. Barry Gurland notes:

> Suicide kills the individual, blights those close to the victim, frustrates the professional care system, and indicts the social environment that allowed it to occur. Thus, the psychological and moral consequences of suicide are just as important a concern as its lethal nature.

In discussing the role of the community agency in serving the mentally frail elderly, Sophie Weiner presents some important insights and a very apt comment:

> I see some elderly as frightened creatures living in isolated caves. In order to be helpful we must be ready to enter their caves to empathize with them in their fear and pain, and attempt to help them if possible to tame the wild beasts that they think they see around them.

A Challenge to the Long-Term Care System

Not only is the acting-out older person a challenge to the professional and the agency but also to the long-term care system as it exists today. This group or set of groups impacts on the various service settings that are components of the existing continuum of care for older persons, e.g., the adult home, the nursing home, the acute hospital, the senior center, the home care project, the protective services agency, the family. The impact of the "hard-to-manage" elderly on the senior center was explored previously in a study conducted by the National Institute of Senior Centers of the National Council on the Aging (1979). Center personnel are often on the front lines in serving this population. Many of these center staff feel ill-equipped to deal with this group in senior centers as their programs do not contain psychiatric components and these clients are stigmatized. Likewise, home care personnel do not have needed psychiatric resources available.

The acting-out elderly may frustrate institutional personnel as well. The multiplicity of problems often defy classification into the current levels of institutional care available. The older person with early dementia, for example, may be too physically intact to qualify for skilled nursing care, yet too mentally impaired to be placed in a less supervised setting such as health-related or intermediate care facility, where he/she is required to function with some independence in the basic activities of daily living. Even if he/she is accepted into an intermediate care facility, he/she may not be suitable for that setting and may require a spectrum of added services just to maintain his/her limited level of functioning within that institution. There is no third-party reimbursement for these added services, and they, therefore, usually are not available.

The second section of this book includes a study which explores the impact of the placement of large numbers of deinstitutionalized patients in adult homes or domiciliary care facilities. The study aptly demonstrated that although the domiciliary care facility is not considered in any statistical analyses as a long-term care facility and is staffed for only minimal supportive supervision, it is, in fact, a long-term institution for a considerable number of hard-to-place elderly. This study demonstrated the need for psychiatric and other supportive services to maintain the residents of adult homes at their maximum level of function in this less restrictive, community-based setting and to diminish the need for repeated hospitalization of ex-mental patients. Models are currently being developed to serve deinstitutionalized patients more effectively. It must be noted, however, that the management of patients with behavioral problems is not an issue that is unique to domiciliary care facilities. Skilled nursing facilities and intermediate care facilities are not equipped for acting-out patients either. The physical plant is designed to serve physically ill persons with relatively limited mobility. Although there is tremendous variation among facilities, the staff is generally geared toward serving a physically ill population. Psychiatric services are often minimal, and staff has little or no training in behavioral interventions.

Now that we have looked at the question of who are the acting-out elderly, let us focus our attention on where they may be encountered.

Where Are the Acting-Out Elderly?

Ninety-five percent of the elderly reside in the community on a given day. Thus, despite prevailing stereotypes, only 5% of older persons are institutionalized at any given time. Institutions which are included in these statistics include long-term mental hospital units, nursing homes, and veterans hospital long-stay wards. How many institutionalized elderly fall into the category of the "acting-out" is almost impossible to determine. It is reported that at least 60% of all nursing home residents carry some diagnosis of mental impairment (Butler and Lewis, 1982). Interestingly, adult homes and other similar domiciliary care facilities are not considered in the statistical compilations about the elderly in institutions despite the fact that these facilities are home to a large number of older persons.[1]

Furthermore, for every nursing home resident with a functional impairment, there are between one and 2.5 persons of similar impairment who are residing outside of institutions (Vladeck, 1980). The scope of the problem of the acting-out elderly is not inconsequential and is by no means limited to institutions.

Frailty, vulnerability, and risk for a variety of problems increase with advancing age in the elderly. The Federal Council on Aging (1978) has advocated that the "group of elderly beginning at age 75 should be viewed as a target population with special needs by reason of their vulnerability." This vulnerability results from decreased physical and emotional capacities. Strained finances may be a contribut-

---

[1] Actual statistics seem to be unclear. The U.S. Dept. of HEW Report on Vital & Health Statistics, The Inpatient Health Facilities, as reported from the 1976 INFI Survey Series 14, No. 23, indicates that there are 240,773 beds in 7,051 surveyed personal and other care homes. Other estimates are much higher.

ing factor in many cases, as are diminished social supports (Federal Council on Aging, 1978). As much as vulnerability does in fact increase with advancing age, it must be cautioned that chronological age by itself is not a good criterion for service need. Functional status is more appropriate. Current estimates are that almost 40% of the elderly are limited to some extent in carrying out major activities of daily living (Harris, 1978). This statistic certainly does not tell the whole story. In order to appreciate the complexity of determining a definition of a target population, it might be well to look at various other statistics.

- 86% of the elderly suffer from one or more chronic illnesses, with varying levels of impairment ranging from mild discomfort to incapacitation (Butler and Lewis, 1982).
- 5% of the elderly are severely incapacitated by dementia; another 10% are mildly to moderately affected (Katzman and Karasu, 1975).
- 3 million elderly are estimated to be in serious need of mental health services (Federal Council on Aging, 1979).
- 6% of the elderly are estimated to be alcoholic; however, this may be an underestimate (Mishara and Kastenbaum, 1980).
- Approximately one-third of the elderly live alone, which may make them more at risk for institutionalization in times of crisis (Federal Council on Aging, 1978).
- 14% of the elderly live below the poverty level (Federal Council on Aging, 1978).
- 25% of suicides in the United States are committed by persons 65 or over. This is disproportionate to the fact that the elderly comprise only 11% of the general population (Federal Council on Aging, 1978). In 1982, we can expect that more than 6,000 older persons will commit suicide (Gurland, 1981).

It has been estimated that there are 36,000 homeless men and women living in the streets of New York City alone. No estimates are available regarding how many of these people are elderly. Many are discharged mental patients. The problem is not indigenous to New York; similar statistics are available for other cities (Baxter and Hopper, 1981).

What does this all mean? None of these categories is mutually exclusive. Essentially, there are large numbers of older persons with a multiplicity of overlapping and interrelated problems and with what appears to be an array of service needs.

Services

Most of this population, however, is not very well serviced, partly due to the system and partly due to their problems. Many often do not fit within the narrowly defined categories of the existing service network. For example, despite the increasingly widespread recognition of the importance of home care services for the mentally frail elderly, one survey found that only 3% of home services to persons of all ages were designated as serving mental health needs (Berkman, 1977). Moreover, if they are eligible for services, they may be resistant to accepting them. Should they accept services initially, an ongoing relationship may be difficult to maintain due to their poor socialization skills. When they are engaged in treatment, they may be an enigma and perhaps even a source of frustration to the professionals who are trying to help them.

Nonetheless, various attempts are being made. Program models have been developed for specific target subgroups of the hard-to-manage population. Some of these models are discussed in the fourth section from both theoretical and pragmatic viewpoints.

Implications

Given current demographic projections, it is quite likely that the numbers of acting-out elderly will increase dramatically in the coming years. If these groups are difficult to deal with now, they will most likely be more problematic in the future. Steps should be taken immediately to recognize the extent of the problem. Moreover, training should be provided for the helping professionals who must deal with these clients. Furthermore, the service delivery system must be modified to accommodate the needs of these persons.

This volume and the conference on which it is based are viewed as beginning steps in delineating and ultimately dealing with these important issues.

The conference was held in New York City at the Albert Einstein College of Medicine in June 1980. This training conference was sponsored by the Albert Einstein College of Medicine Long Term Care Gerontology Center, the Columbia University Center on Geriatrics and Gerontology, and the Center on Aging of Fordham University. Approximately 150 persons from a variety of disciplines attended, and their concerns and feedback are reflected in the papers contained herein.

The scope of the day's proceedings was rather broad and encompassed attention to questions of who is this population, where are they, and how do you handle them?

Part II

IDENTIFYING THE ACTING-OUT ELDERLY

Prologue

This section contains two very different papers. The first is an anecdotal, highly personal account of the experiences of the head of a major community service agency, in which she describes the range of cases which are encountered. The second is a preliminary report on a statistical study of deinstitutionalized mental patients in proprietary homes for adults, a singular and unique type of setting.

Though these papers are very different, they are related in that the acting-out elderly are not a homogeneous group, and where they live, i.e., community vs. institution, probably relates more to circumstances such as prior family relationships and encounters with the service delivery system, than to current functional status.

How Does the Community Agency Deal with the Acting-Out Elderly on a Day-to-Day Basis?

Sophie Weiner, MSW

In trying to answer the question, how does the community agency deal with the hard-to-manage or acting-out elderly on a day-to-day basis, I would have to say, "with a good deal of courage and commitment." Although there are a great many feelings of frustration, helplessness, shock, revulsion, and burnout, these are counterbalanced by feelings of satisfaction and the joy of accomplishment and of work well done.

Before I discuss how, let me briefly describe who. The acting-out elderly person may be depicted graphically as a "suffering senior," i.e., living in an abandoned building where he or she is without electricity, heat, or food and prey to addicts, or in less extreme cases, disheveled, disoriented, and in need of medical attention, or forgetful or confused and in need of household help or relocation, or an aggressive street person. The problems are many and varied. To quote Helen Turner Burr:

> Of all the misfortunes which people suffer in their old age, mental impairments are among the most numerous and baffling. Mental impairment, an omen of personal dissolution, falls like a curse on the victim who experiences it and as a blight to those who witness it. Of all the barriers to functioning as whole social beings, decline of our mental faculties is the most dangerous, since it attacks the organ of thinking and personality, our central identity as individuals; it may wipe out the person who was, and reveal a stranger. (Burr, 1976)

Sophie Weiner is Bronx Borough Director, Jewish Association of Services for the Aged, New York, NY.

The needs are often not clear. The older person him/herself often may not realize that there is a problem, and he or she may, therefore, not seek help for something that may seem obvious to others. Says Sister Jean Golden:

> Society functions on the assumption that anyone who is really ill will seek some type of medical assistance, but with the elderly who are frightened of agencies and often too infirm to get to a doctor or clinic the assumption is a fallacy. (Golden, 1976)

Often, the person does not seek help but rather may come to the attention of friends, family, or neighbors.

The First Contact

Our first contact, therefore, is often through a third party who contacts our telephone information or intake service. The caller may be a relative, friend, social agency, hospital, clergyman, or building superintendent. Sometimes the relative or some concerned community member will actually come to the agency office. Only very occasionally will the elderly person him/herself call or come to the agency. The intake worker may feel helpless and overwhelmed by the complexity of the problems presented and usually seeks supervisory assistance in devising a plan.

The Home Visit: A First Step in Assessment

Our first step in intervention almost always involves making a home visit. To develop an appropriate plan, I feel it is necessary to assess the person in the context of his/her environment. I see some impaired elderly as frightened creatures living in isolated caves. In order to be helpful, we must be ready to enter their caves to empathize with them in their fear and pain, and attempt to help them if possible to tame the wild beasts that they think they see around them. We must do this despite the disbelief and revulsion we may experience upon making the home visit.

Accepting the Client as He/She Is

We try to understand that no matter how bizarre the behavior may appear, the aged person is defending him/herself against further disintegration and trying to communicate a message to the world. We try to avoid being judgmental and accept the client as he/she is. We try to think of our clients as more than "a paranoid man" or "a dirty, smelly, old woman." Despite the unpleasant outward appearance, creativity, humor, warmth, and other parts of the personality still remain. We let the client know that we are ready to become parent surrogates while still searching for his/her remaining strengths. One of the methods of gaining the trust of the client is to do something concrete for him or her and accept him or her as he/she is.

I would like to illustrate this with some case histories.

> Mr. B. suffered from dementia and many physical ailments. He told me that they were threatening to shoot him at sunrise, but he would fool them because he never got up that early. While I made it a policy not to lend money to patients, I broke this rule for Mr. B. He usually would borrow one dollar, stating that he would not be around long enough to repay me. I assured him that he would, showing him I trusted him and believed in his continued existence. He always paid it back promptly.

> Mr. C., a client of our agency, was by his own description a street person. Sometimes he lived in deteriorated rooming houses or slept in abandoned cars or buildings. He found warmth and acceptance at a local senior center, but they had difficulty tolerating his filthy appearance and lice and, at times, his behavior. Our social worker went to the Center regularly and washed his hair. He would then eat with him at his favorite coffee shop. When he needed a period of hospitalization at a psychiatric hospital, he trusted this social worker enough to go to the hospital with him and be admitted voluntarily.

Ms. D., a deinstitutionalized psychiatric patient, is now residing in the community and is followed conjointly by a state hospital worker and a staff person from our agency. There are periods when she has difficulty maintaining herself. On occasion our worker has cooked breakfast for the client when her disturbance has prevented her from preparing her own meals.

These cases are illustrative of the variety of cases that are encountered. Helen Turner Burr's observation regarding the impaired elderly comes to mind:

> Though impaired older persons are all impelled by the same need to find help in order to survive, they may act in very different ways to do so. They may choose alternately to force, shame or persuade us into taking their part. Those who try to arouse sympathy for weakness or helplessness may appear to us instead irritatingly apathetic and unwilling to cope with the simplest tasks. On the other hand some who wish to try to disguise their inner weakness by annoying or offensive complaining, blustering, commanding or attacking us, intending only to make us respect them because they are "strong." (Burr, 1976, p. 109)

Getting through the outer facade is not always easy.

Helping the Family to Cope

When the acting-out client has a family close at hand, the challenge of our job is to work with them to aid them in dealing with their aged relative. This objective of our agency has been stated succinctly by David Soyer:

> Our purpose becomes that of helping the family cope in a way that is consistent not with some objective sense of right or wrong, but with the family's own needs, its life patterns, its sense of worth. Whatever the solution it chooses, the family should be left with some degree of comfort and some degree of integrity, even if it

must choose a course that is really not in the best interests of the older person himself. (Soyer, 1972)

Sometimes this is easier said than done. Family members often engage in denial, for to face the fact that an omnipotent parent is failing is too painful. In my first job with the aged, a client reported to me that over "250 tenants had been gassed to death by their landlords." Her family denied that there were any psychiatric problems and attributed her difficulty to a gall bladder condition.

Other times, routine situations escalate into crises due to overwhelming demands on family or other caretakers rather than a deterioration of the patient's condition. Richard Moryez finds this characteristic of dementing illness:

> Oftentimes problems presented by dementing older individuals are allowed to assume crisis proportions, partly because of a lack of understanding by individuals in caretaker positions, and also partly because of a lack of resources in the community. Most emergencies concerning older persons are not generated by any immediate deterioration in the patients' conditions, but result from unbearable escalation of pressure on their family or other support givers. (Moryez, 1980)

When the family finds itself under stress, old conflicts and wounds reemerge, and seemingly buried rivalries can surface. Often the disturbed parent did not provide much nurturance to the children, and to ask them to assume what Margaret Blenkner called "filial maturity" can seem like too much of a burden. The conflict becomes especially painful when the need for institutionalization arises and a decision must be made. To "put one's parent away" for the rest of his/her life can arouse unbearable guilt. The idea of the "dumping" of elderly persons by families has proven untrue in my experience. The adult children feel squeezed by a three-generation crunch, their own needs, those of their children, and the demands of their parents. Many relatives have struggled with the problem for a long time before they finally seek help from a social agency such as ours.

Our agency, in essence, offers to share the burden with

the family and enables them to find their own strengths. Some of the services offered include: counselling to examine familial relationships, interpretation of the disturbed relative's behavior, housekeeping services, financial assistance, assessing the need for other services, and referral as appropriate. When placement is indicated, we help the family to make a decision to effect it and then to implement it, as is illustrated by the following case:

> Mrs. M. and her brother Mr. T. came to me to seek help for their aged mother and stepfather, Mr. and Mrs. S. Mrs. S. had been discharged from a state hospital, the stepfather was mildly disoriented. At first we tried keeping them at home for several months, with the aid of a homemaker but it was unsuccessful. Mrs. S. would fight with the homemakers and eventually throw them out. She called her daughter at all hours of the night accusing her of many different crimes. Even though her daughter gave a great deal of herself, she could do nothing right. I liked Mrs. S., and her intelligence came through despite her paranoid behavior. When I told her this, she beamed and said, "it's not so much that you like me but you understand me." A decision was made to place the couple. It was felt they could manage in a nursing home, and I helped the family locate a suitable one. They asked that I accompany them on the day of placement. It was a sad day for the family and me. While the couple were packing the few meager belongings they were permitted at the institution, Mrs. S. Said, "I worked all my life for a house not a nursing home." I obtained a picture of the nursing home and showed it to both of them. When we arrived, I helped the couple, along with their children, to get settled and to orient themselves to the setting.

While I cannot say they made a perfect adjustment, my participation in the placement process and subsequent visits after placement appeared to have a positive impact on Mr. and Mrs. S. and their children during a chaotic time in their lives.

Seeking Out Other Support Systems

Families and agencies cannot do it all. It is essential to seek out the support systems that the client may have already developed, strengthen them whenever possible, and look for new ones. The client may prefer a friend or neighbor to an agency. On the other hand, we must also be aware of the systems that may be potentially harmful or destructive to the aged person. The client's vulnerability and confusion can make him/her prey to those who, under the guise of helping, may steal his/her money and possessions. The neighbor who is cashing checks for the client may be pocketing all or most of it. In one situation, a friendly neighborhood TV repair man was managing all of the client's finances and exploiting her. While laws to protect the aged are almost nonexistent, agencies sometimes can be helpful. The Bronx Senior Citizens Robbery Unit has also become involved in some of these situations and has been very effective.

More commonly than their being destructive forces however, we have found that friends, neighbors, local merchants, and superintendents have been invaluable as caretakers and community supports. Countless numbers of these people are responsible for helping the frail elderly person to function in the community on a day-to-day basis. They call us when they no longer handle the problems alone. Often we can assist them and develop a partnership which enables the frail elderly person to remain in the community. A case comes to mind:

> Mr. L., a client of our Crisis Intervention Unit, was disoriented, incontinent, and severely malnourished. He resided in a housing project and during the team's visit, several concerned neighbors were present. The neighbor who had been most involved, Mr. H., was of a different race and totally different ethnic background. The team feared that Mr. H. would require hospitalization but hesitated. It was suggested that someone offer Mr. L. the food that Mr. H. brought in on a roll, which Mr. L. almost devoured, and the neighbors clapped and cheered. We were able to hire

Mr. H. as his housekeeper, and when a conservator was appointed, he continued to employ Mr. H. Several years have elapsed, and although Mr. L. still has problems, to my knowledge, he is still in the community.

Professional Collaboration

Agencies work with other agencies. Agencies also need a support network. We seek out and utilize other agencies, for we cannot do it alone. Hot lunches may be the only nutrition received by the aged person, and we work closely with a broad spectrum of health and social agencies who may provide home delivered meals for our frail clients.

Another necessary component is medical backup. Finding a doctor to make home visits is almost impossible, but several years ago one of our case aides, to whom I am still grateful, found a dedicated physician who is still working with us. His ability to hospitalize our clients, when necessary, has saved lives. When state hospitals refused to admit geriatric patients except under some very special circumstances, we found some private psychiatric facilities willing to work with us, and we continue to use them.

When you ask how do we deal on a day-to-day basis, I say we manage. We try to assist a hard-to-manage, frail population who need supportive services in order to remain in the community. Our approach is pragmatic and has been described as follows:

> It is perhaps the lack of any institutional base, the overwhelming demand for help, and our location in a city where services of all kinds are fragmented and make bureaucratic by the very size of the city, that have led to a pragmatic approach in an attempt to search and scratch to bring something human into situations for which there are often no real answers. (Soyer, 1972, p. 52)

While we do not have the solutions to all problems, we are right there in the community working in the front lines to advocate for our clients and attempt to make some positive difference in the quality of their lives. The fact that we can do this and that we can persist in doing this gives us a sense of purpose and accomplishment which makes the job personally satisfying.

Behavior Problems Encountered in Adult Homes

Alvin Mesnikoff, MD
David Wilder, PhD

The private proprietary home for adults (PPHA or adult home) has become a major residential resource for the deinstitutionalized mentally ill. After 1968, when the New York State Department of Mental Hygiene began its major effort at deinstitutionalization, large numbers of chronic mental patients were referred to adult homes. Private entrepreneurs, aware of the need for residential facilities for the thousands of patients being discharged from New York State hospitals, were encouraged to respond to this need by the availability of government-sponsored mortgage programs that encouraged the building of new facilities that would qualify for Medicaid funding.

The adult home was designed to provide residential care for those frail, aged, and/or disabled adults who required supportive services in a protective environment and was part of the continuum for the long-range care for the chronically ill. It provides 24-hour residential care to persons who do not require continual medical or nursing care, but who are unable to live independently and require supportive services. It provides room and board, housekeeping services, personal care services, supervision, and other nonmedical services to insure safety and well-being. In the beginning, monitoring and regulation by the New York State Board of Social Welfare did not keep up with the needs of the deinstitutionalized population. Numerous investigations reported poor conditions in the adult homes and that residents received inadequate supervision and care. Various attempts were made to upgrade the care in these facilities, but it was not until 1978 in connection with the introduction of the Community Support System program (CSS) that a more systematic approach was begun (see Part IV). Prior to establishment of this program, an attempt was made to survey systematically the population of adult homes. Preliminary data from this survey are discussed in this paper.

Method

Data for this survey were obtained from the Client Assessment forms designed for the CSS program. At the time these data were obtained from the New York State Office of Mental Health, there were 1,900 residents of PPHAs included in the data system. Since there were approximately 20,000 residents in PPHAs in New York State at that time, these data represent about 9% of the total resident population of these facilities. These data include residents from a wide-range of PPHAs throughout the state, but it should be noted that this is not a random sample, and some facilities and areas are not represented at all. Hence, the figures reported should be regarded as preliminary and ungeneralizable. Nevertheless, it should be emphasized that these data are illustrative of many characteristics of the PPHAs and the mixes of populations they serve.

To reduce the data on behavior problems to a more manageable format, eight scales were assembled to represent relevant problem areas for PPHA residents. The scales were constructed by combining items on the Client Assessment forms that had face validity and were strongly related statistically. The individual items comprising each scale and the methods of scoring are available upon request. The eight conceptual problem areas are:

- physical health
- inactivity and social withdrawal
- personal grooming and care
- functional level
- acting-out behavior
- antisocial behavior
- drug and alcohol abuse
- danger to self or others.

Findings

The aged are overrepresented in the PPHA. Thirty-seven percent of the residents in the sample were aged 65 or older compared with 11% in the United States population. Persons who are known to be former mental patients comprised about half of the sample, and the vast majority of these are chronic patients who had been hospitalized for six months or longer (Table 1). But similar to the population at large, the proportion of males and females are about equal among those under 65, and females comprise 60% of the over-65 group.

The physical health of the vast majority of adult home residents is excellent or very good as measured by our scale (Table 2), but the differences between the two age groups are substantial. Eighty-two percent of the under-65 group have "excellent" or "very good" health compared with just 58% of the older residents. These age differences are in keeping with the findings of general health surveys that consistently show that while the majority of people over 65 exhibit good health, much higher proportions of those over 65 have health problems than those under 65.

TABLE 1

PPHA Residents by Age
and Known Former Patient Status

Age	Known Patient Status			Other
	6+ Months	3 x 10 days	3+ Months in 2 years	
<65	41%	3%	3%	53%
(1131)	(458)	(30)	(39)	(603)
≥65	41%	---	2%	57%
(652)	(269)		(10)	(373)

TABLE 2

Percent of PPHA Residents in 3 Scoring Categories on Physical Health Scale
(Sample numbers in parentheses)

Age	Physical Health		
	Excellent or very good	Good	Fair or Poor
<65 (1034)	82% (844)	14% (148)	4% (42)
≥65 (572)	58% (331)	32% (181)	10% (60)

In contrast with physical health, functional levels of only a small minority of residents are classified as "good." But again there are marked differences between the two age groups, with 67% of the under-65 group scoring as "fair" and "poor" compared with 83% of the older group (Table 3). Items in this scale refer to such matters as ability to use public transportation, to perform household chores, and to manage medications independently.

Slightly more than half of the PPHA residents scored "good" on the two-item personal grooming and care scale, 50% of the younger and 48% of the older group (Table 4). Hence it appears that the functional levels of residents and their personal grooming and care are lower than one would expect on the basis of their physical health scores alone.

Consistent with this pattern are the scores of the Inactivity and Social Withdrawal Scale. Only 36% of the younger and 31% of the older scored "good" on this scale (Table 5). (This scale contains the single most frequently checked item, "Does nothing most days.")

The profile from scale scores up to this point is one of PPHA residents who are generally physically healthy, but who have high levels of functional disability, difficulties

TABLE 3

Percent of PPHA Residents in 3 Scoring Categories
on Functional Level Scale
(Sample numbers in parentheses)

Age	Functional Level		
	Good	Fair	Poor
<65	33%	57%	10%
(1131)	(372)	(647)	(112)
≥65	17%	65%	18%
(652)	(113)	(421)	(118)

TABLE 4

Percent of PPHA Residents in 3 Scoring Categories
on Personal Grooming and Care Scale
(Sample numbers in parentheses)

Age	Personal Grooming and Care		
	Good	Fair	Poor
<65	59%	34%	6%
(1182)	(700)	(406)	(76)
≥65	48%	45%	7%
(683)	(327)	(311)	(45)

with personal grooming and care, and considerable inactivity and social withdrawal.

Turning to the more disruptive forms of behavior, a very different profile emerges. Table 6 indicates that acting-out

TABLE 5

Percent of PPHA Residents in 3 Scoring Categories on Inactivity and Social Withdrawal Scale
(Sample numbers in parentheses)

Age	Inactivity and Social Withdrawal		
	Good	Fair	Poor
<65 (1117)	36% (402)	48% (537)	16% (178)
≥65 (665)	31% (203)	56% (373)	13% (89)

TABLE 6

Percent of PPHA Residents in 3 Scoring Categories on Acting-Out Behavior Scale
(Sample numbers in parentheses)

Age	Acting-Out Behavior		
	Good	Fair	Poor
<65 (1155)	87% (1008)	12% (138)	1% (9)
≥65 (642)	95% (610)	5% (31)	1% (1)

behavior (such things as trouble at school or work, causing complaints in the household or community, losing temper or self-control, bizarre or unusual behavior, etc.) is scored as "good" (not present) for 87% of the under-65 group and for 95% of the older group.

Antisocial behavior (i.e., trouble with the law, destroying

property or stealing property) is not present among 94% and 98% of the younger and older groups respectively as shown in Table 7.

Drug and alcohol abuse are scored as "none" for 89% of the younger and 96% of the older groups as shown in Table 8.

TABLE 7

Percent of PPHA Residents in 3 Scoring Categories on Antisocial Behavior Scale
(Sample numbers in parentheses)

Age	Antisocial Behavior		
	None	Mild	Serious
<65 (1105)	94% (1034)	5% (51)	2% (20)
≥65 (632)	98% (618)	2% (10)	1% (4)

TABLE 8

Percent of PPHA Residents in 3 Scoring Categories on Drug and Alcohol Abuse Scale
(Sample numbers in parentheses)

Age	Drug and Alcohol Abuse		
	None	Mild	Serious
<65 (1118)	89% (995)	6% (69)	5% (54)
≥65 (632)	95% (599)	4% (26)	1% (7)

TABLE 9

Percent of PPHA Residents in 3 Scoring Categories on Danger to Self or Others Scale
(Sample numbers in parentheses)

Age	Danger to Self or Others		
	None	Mild	Serious
<65	90%	8%	2%
(1148)	(1029)	(92)	(27)
≥65	96%	3%	1%
(649)	(625)	(20)	(4)

Being a danger to oneself or others is judged not present in 96% of the older group as shown in Table 9.

Discussion

It is evident from the data presented that the adult home population is heterogeneous with regard to age and sex, but that there is an overrepresentation of older persons in the population mix. The majority of residents exhibit functional incapacities, social withdrawal, and inactivity. Large proportions have difficulty in grooming and personal care as well. Only a small minority of residents are reported as acting-out, abusing drugs or alcohol, behaving antisocially, or being a danger to themselves or to others. While the numbers are small, it is, of course, these behaviors that are the most difficult to handle and present significant management problems in the homes.

Acting-out, antisocial behaviors, and drug and alcohol abuse were consistently found less often among the elderly than among the younger residents, while inactivity, social withdrawal, and poor personal grooming were more frequently found among the elderly. These findings corroborate divergent needs among a heterogeneous population and an indication for the development of appropriate approaches. This need for varying strategies is a challenge to the helping professionals who service these facilities and to the agencies who fund them at a single rate rather than according to resident mix.

On the other hand, this variability of resident mix in adult homes provides an excellent opportunity for learning more about whether heterogeneous groups can support one another within a single setting and can thus improve the quality of life within that context.

Epilogue

COUNSELING CONSULTANTS

Ms. Weiner's article is descriptive in nature and gives the reader a feeling for the types of cases that present themselves to the community agency and for the multiplicity of complex problems that must be dealt with in devising appropriate interventions. One can also get a sense of the great lengths to which a worker (or an agency) must often go to serve these clients.

Despite the need for individualized intervention plans, certain general principles are apparent in this approach:

1. *Client/worker relationship* must be developed. Worker must often see the client at home and work with him/her "where he/she is at," despite a bizarre or unpleasant life-style.
2. *Working with families.* Families usually do not call upon agencies until they are overwhelmed by circumstances. The community agency must often support family members to maintain their caretaking activities.
3. *Working with other support systems,* e.g., friends, neighbors, shopkeepers, to help maintain the frail person in his/her preferred environment.
4. *Working collaboratively with other agencies and disciplines* which are capable of meeting needs that the primary agency cannot fill.

This community agency tends to take a pragmatic, nontreatment-oriented approach. It is evident that this approach requires infinite flexibility and openness on the part of not only the line worker but also the agency administration. The net result is probably a less restrictive environment for the clients, some of whom might, under other circumstances, be institutionalized.

The paper by Drs. Mesnikoff and Wilder provides some statistical data regarding behavior problems encountered in adult homes.

The major problems of the elderly in these settings are functional inability, poor physical health, inactivity, social withdrawal, and poor personal care. While the rates were low overall, more acting-out was found among the younger residents of adult homes.

Only half of adult home residents were discharged mental patients.

The reader can get a feel for the fact that many of the stereotypes of the adult home are erroneous.

In fact, based on the data presented and on the relative rate of reimbursement, one might ask whether this is an appropriate setting for the elderly. Attempts at developing a service model for enriching this environment are discussed in Part IV.

Part III

SOME FORMS OF ACTING-OUT BEHAVIOR

Prologue

This section contains papers on two topics which are relevant to any discussion of acting-out. Dr. Ruth Bennett discusses the socially isolated elderly, a group without contacts in late life, who may or may not have been isolated all their lives. These people tend to adjust poorly to new situations—institutionalization for example. At times one might ask whether they are "acting out" or "acting in," e.g., withdrawing and isolating themselves.

Dr. Barry Gurland provides an overview of suicide and the elderly, dealing with a problem that is probably the most difficult for professionals to face. Despite our best efforts, if a person is determined to end his/her life, he/she may succeed. And when he/she does, it leaves an indelible impression on all of us. Dr. Gurland puts the problem in perspective providing an epidemiologic overview, looks at the relationship between suicide and other variables (such as illness and mental illness), and discusses a broad-based approach.

Those who are forced (or involuntary) isolates are undoubtedly at greater risk for suicide.

The Socially Isolated Elderly

Ruth Bennett, PhD

Social isolation is a complex issue in the elderly. It is possible that older people who are socially isolated in the community, either involuntarily or because they have voluntarily disengaged themselves, will be stressed upon entry to an institution or a senior center when they are forced to interact with others. This process may resemble relocation stress, and that stress may be induced by recognition on the part of the older person that he/she is behaving in ways that are offensive to others. It is possible that stress can occur at any point in the course of one's career as a member of a senior center or institution for a variety of reasons—not the least of which are losses of relatives and friends inside and outside the senior center, losses which are occurring simultaneously with participation in a center or institution.

The background for these ideas based on some of our early research will be reviewed. Beginning with a study of 100 case records of the Jewish Home and Hospital for the Aged (JHHA) in 1957 and a related direct survey of 100 elderly residents, it was found that residents who experienced isolation before entering a home had difficulty becoming socialized. In a series of studies, we examined the relationship between social isolation, morale, social adjustment, mental status, and cognitive functioning. The findings were that social isolation has a negative impact on the institutionalized elderly. (These studies are described in detail in Bennett, 1980.) While the factor of social isolation was identified as having a negative impact on adjustment, other researchers have sought to describe other factors which have stressing effects after relocation of the elderly person.

Ruth Bennett is Deputy Director, Center for Geriatrics and Gerontology, Columbia University.

In our first study, which was conducted by directly interviewing residents of the JHHA, we found the following distribution of social isolation: Table 1 shows that 45% of 100 consecutive admissions to JHHA were lifelong (or, perhaps, voluntary) isolates.

These were people who often described themselves as loners, who had a life-style that went along with that description, and who might have been content to steer clear of people for the rest of their lives had they not, for one reason or another, come into an institution where they were forced to interact. As we now know from recent national institutional surveys, about 50% of the elderly in institutions may fall into this category. Many of them have no living relatives, had never married, had no children, or had experienced a combination of these factors. Given the fact that institutionalization for social reasons (such as isolation) is nearly impossible in New York these days, some of these people may now be turning up in senior centers.

Fourteen percent of the original group studied was invol-

TABLE 1

Relation between Pattern of Isolation and Socialization at Two Months

(1957 Jewish Home and Hospital Sample of 100)

Isolation Pattern	Combination of Adulthood & Past Month Isolation Scores		Socialization at Two Months	
	Adulthood Isolation	Past Month or Pre-Entry Isolation	N	% Above Median
Nonisolate	Not isolated	Not isolated	31	77
Early isolate	Isolated	Not isolated	10	50
Involuntary isolate	Not isolated	Isolated	14	36
Voluntary or lifelong isolate	Isolated	Isolated	45	29
			n=100	

untarily isolated, i.e., they had interacted socially with friends and relatives early in life but had lost their social contacts in old age. This group has been found to be responsive to social and other programs offered in a number of successive studies (Bennett, 1980; Bennett and Cook, 1980). Certainly, they would be happy to be in a center but might remain somewhat desocialized. Ten percent were early isolates who may never have married or had children early in life but who were not without contacts late in life. Finally, 31% were never isolated.

As you can see from Table 1, this last pattern of isolation was highly related to becoming socialized in the institution, that is, learning its rules and norms by 2 months. Table 1 also shows that the least socialized group were the lifelong or voluntary isolates.

Contrary to expectation, socialization was not affected by duration of social isolation alone. Table 1 shows that when individuals who were relatively isolated in adulthood but not in old age were compared with those who were isolated for the first time as a concomitant of aging; the latter had greater difficulty becoming socialized which suggested that there may be critical periods for desocialization, as well as resocialization. We also found that all isolation was bad as far as its effects on socialization were concerned. The score differences between nonisolates and the group next in line were greater than between any other two groups. While the voluntary or lifelong isolates (perhaps some were mentally disordered) did worst of all, it was not much worse than involuntary isolates. However, the gap widens between involuntary isolation and early isolation and widens most between early isolation and no isolation at all.

Findings in Table 2 show that people who experienced isolation before entering a home for the aged had significantly greater difficulty becoming socialized than those who were not isolated.

The relation between socialization and isolation was greater than the relation between isolation and any of the three components of adjustment, thus supporting a hypothesis that desocialization, or the inability to perceive social cues currently, was an intervening factor which mediated between isolation experienced prior to entry and subse-

TABLE 2

Rank-Order (Rho) Correlations between Isolation, Socialization, and Adjustment after one, two, and six months of residence in a home

Isolation and socialization	One Month				Two Months				Six Month Total Adjustment
	Soc.	Int.	Eval.	Conf.	Soc.	Int.	Eval.	Conf.	
Adulthood	.23*	.21*	.20	.00	.22*	.23*	.04	.11	.09
Pre-Entry	.27+	.16	.07	.02	.27+	.22*	.08	.13	.19*
Socialization (one month)		.51+⁺	.26+	.08	.79+⁺	.50+⁺	.12	.02	.32+
Socialization (two months)						.48+⁺	.10	-.04	.26+

*P <.05
+P <.01
+⁺ <.001

quent poor adjustment. Early or rapid socialization, rather than socialization *per se*, related best to adjustment, i.e., those who learned the ropes in the first month adjusted better than those who subsequently learned them.

What does this mean? It seems to mean that if you have not interacted with others for long periods of time and then, either voluntarily or involuntarily, enter a social setting, you will have trouble learning the ropes, and this may mean you will behave in ways which will cause you difficulties with institutional staff, residents, staff of senior centers, or other clients of senior centers. These findings, based on direct studies, were consistent with those of our first study which had been based on case records only.

In 1957 we began a study of "Mental Disorders of the Senium" at the Jewish Home and Hospital for the Aged (JHHA) financed by a small grant from NIMH. We examined 100 case records of residents who were transferred to a mental hospital from JHHA and those who were not. Fifty residents of the Home who were transferred were compared to controls matched for age, sex, and length of residence who remained in the Home. The findings showed that social isolation experienced prior to entering the Home was related to inability to get along with staff members and other residents, a sign of maladjustment which often resulted in a transfer to a mental hospital. The factors which predicted to transfer were low socioeconomic status in childhood, negative attitudes towards the Home on initial admission, and being labeled a management problem. Neither psychiatric diagnosis nor psychiatric history was related to transfer to a mental hospital—probably because at that time the Home screened out persons with a known psychiatric history or diagnosis.

Nearly 20 years after our first study at the JHHA, a study of case records of 100 persons was conducted at JHHA by Rodstein, Savitsky, and Starkman (1976) on initial adjustment to a long-term care institution. They found the following:

> The aged persons most likely to have initial adjustment difficulties usually had poor capacity for interpersonal relationships, were socially isolated, were either single or divorced, had dependent personality, had severe chronic brain syndrome, had a negative or ambivalent attitude toward admission and often had been referred for psychiatric evaluation before admission. (p. 65)

Both the similarities and the differences in the findings of the two sets of case record-based studies, conducted nearly 20 years apart, are of interest. First, the similarities: Isolation and negative attitudes on admission continued to predict to poor adjustment initially, and some of those who were admitted improved with increased length of stay. Second, the differences: These probably can be accounted for by the changes in the average age on admission (from mid-seventies to mid-eighties in 20 years), by a change in the Home's policy to admit and retain those with psychiatric disorders and histories, and by the change in the Home's psychiatric capabilities which makes it possible for the Home to retain the mentally disordered and does not require that they be transferred to a mental hospital. Presumably the increased capacity to diagnose and treat the mentally ill who become maladjusted accounts in part for the findings reported by Rodstein, Savitsky, and Starkman (1976) that over half of the 50 patients with initial adjustment difficulties reached "a satisfactory level of adaptation during the first six months after admission."

From our early studies it was not clear whether the maladjusted behavior seen in the institutionalized aged was the result of isolation or of mental disorder. Nor did we know if both isolation and maladjustment resulted from mental disorder. Thus, a study of the relations between psychiatric illness, adjustment, and pre-entry isolation was undertaken. Fifty-three successive admissions to the home for the aged who were already studied in earlier research were independently evaluated by Dr. Henry Walton, a British-trained psychiatrist, using a crude standard diagnostic instrument of geriatric mental state to gauge impairment of intellectual ability and presence of functional psychiatric illness. The findings showed no significant relation between isolation experienced prior to entry and mental disorder.

However, some forms of mental disorder did result in extreme maladjustment. Residents suffering from senile and arteriosclerotic dementia were differentiated from those with functional psychiatric disorder by their social adjustment patterns. Those with dementia adjusted to the institutional environment with a sense of subjective satisfaction and in accordance with the institution's expectations. But those with functional psychiatric disorder were unhappy and, in addition to this personal discomfort, did not conform to social rules or live up to the expectations and requirements of other residents.

This supported our earlier suspicion that there were two or possibly more "syndromes" which were related to similarly maladjusted behavior found among the elderly: one was mental disorder; the other may be termed the "isolation-desocialization syndrome" (Gruenberg, 1969). The "isolation-desocialization syndrome" is a process that may be described as follows. An old person in the community becomes first isolated, then desocialized. He enters a home for the aged or some other setting, misperceives the norms, and blunders socially soon after entrance. Others single him out, perhaps as a "troublemaker," and avoid him. He then becomes involved in overt conflict with staff members and/or other residents. Finally, long experience with social isolation would not be as great a handicap to an old person who remains isolated in the community as it would be to one who is forced to adjust socially. However, also presumably, the sequelae of social isolation may be more remediable conditions than sequelae resulting from mental disorders of the senium.

In the next series of studies conducted in the Home and reported in Bennett (1980) we found that isolation diminished cognitive and social performance while interaction stimulated good performance. At one point in our series of studies we looked for the brighter side of social isolation if there was one. We thought isolation may well have some salutary personality effects, possibly resulting in attitudinal independence, in the "rugged individualist" or "old codger" who will do battle against any restraints. This was not found to be the case; in fact, the opposite was true in that isolates were found to be highly persuasible. Later, several graduate students conducted a series of studies aimed at reducing isolation or its impact. In one such study it was found that by friendly visiting, it was possible to have some direct, salutary effects on some social behaviors, such as increasing social interaction, improving grooming, and reducing illness complaints. On follow-up, isolates who had been visited were found to have increased their social interaction scores.

One student conducted a dissertation study and found that isolates are most helped by resocialization programs. This finding has implications for targeting isolates who are most at risk but who can be helped by social programs.

Now, to tie these studies back to relocation stress, which may well be what is observed when a newcomer to an institution or senior center seems to get the wrong message, seems to be desocialized, engages in antisocial and offensive behavior, or in other ways irritates the staff or clients.

Mirotznick's study (1978) of the relocation of patients at the Kingsbrook Jewish Medical Center to a new facility identified 11 sociodemographic variables which mediated the degree of relocation stress patients experienced. (See Table 3.)

TABLE 3

Eleven Sociodemographic Variables which Mediated the Degree
of Relocation Stress Patients Experienced

Five demographic variables found to explain the most variance were:

- Sex
- Marital Status
- Race
- Number of years spent in all hospitals
- Degree of physical handicap

Six sociological variables found to explain the most variance were:

- Macro integration
- Patient knowledge about the relocation
- Micro integration
- Family integration
- Anomia
- Pre and post relocation change in identity

*From Mirotznick, Jerrold S., "A Sociological Analysis of a Relocation Process." Unpublished PhD dissertation, Rutgers, The State University of New Jersey, 1978.

In Table 3 based on Mirotznick's study we see that lack of knowledge about the new setting (lack of socialization), lack of integration with the larger society (macrointegration), lack of integration with peers (microintegration) prior to the move, lack of integration with family, a sense of anomie (alienation, subjective isolation) all contributed to experiencing relocation stress after nursing home patients were moved from an old building to a new one.

Summary and Conclusion

Isolation experienced prior to entry into an institution has a negative effect on the following: socialization (learning of norms) and adjustment defined as participation in activities, evaluation, and conformity to norms. We know from Mirotznick's (1978) study that isolation contributes to relocation stress. The mechanism by which the two are related is not entirely clear. Do signs of lack of socialization and disruptive behavior lead to further isolation which leads to more disruptive behavior? Or is isolation more involuntary (even if it is a life-style experienced over a lifetime, e.g., because one is shy, ugly, or in some other way unacceptable) which pushes one into a life-style which causes a lack of experience and training in learning socially appropriate behavior or becoming adept at reading social cues? Or is it a combination of the two processes? Or are they a consequence of some other process? Whatever the case may be, we know that isolation is handicapping particularly for those who need to learn quickly to interact with others.

It is highly possible that older people who are socially isolated in the community, either involuntarily or because they have voluntarily disengaged themselves, will be stressed upon entry to an institution where they are forced to interact with roommates, table mates, staff members, and other persons.

Lest you should believe we are simply describing findings that have no bearing on the community aged, I would like you to look at Table 4. Table 4 compares a random sample of 389 New York City elderly with 100 consecutive admissions to a home for the aged on the isolation patterns referred to earlier.

As you would expect, there are more lifelong isolates in the institution (45%) than in the community (32%) suggest-

TABLE 4

Distribution on Patterns of Isolation in New York City and at a Home for Aged

Pattern of Isolation	US (N = 389)	JHHA (N = 100)
Lifelong or Voluntary Isolate	32%	45%
Involuntary Isolate	16%	14%
Recent Active (Early Isolate)	19%	10%
Lifelong Active (Nonisolate)	33%	31%

ing that those who have accumulated few social supports over a lifetime end up in institutions while others, perhaps comparably frail but better supported elderly, remain in the community.

Nonetheless, over 30% lifelong isolates in the community aged represents a large number of people, and as our recent findings on the New York City random sample show, many of them are in genuine need of assistance. Senior centers provide us with an opportunity to assist them. Questions for future research are: how much basic resocialization can be done in senior centers, and what is needed to help them do this job?

Conclusion

A consistent finding has been that involuntary or recent isolates are a good group to target for delivery of services and programs. They make use of these programs when they are available and show improvement after such services and programs are delivered. Persons in this category were found to improve after institutionalization as well as after experiencing time-limited therapy. Their counterparts in the community were also found to make greatest use of services. Given scarce resources, such as institutional services and resocialization programs, it might be useful to target the involuntary isolate; he or she will use them and benefit the most from them.

Suicide among the Elderly

Barry J. Gurland, MD, MRCP
Peter S. Cross, MS, MPhil

In this society and culture we are disturbed by suicide more than by most other causes of death and for quite understandable reasons. As professionals in health and social care, our mandate to preserve life and well-being is flouted by the deliberate taking of a life; the conduct of treatment and the morale of staff are upset by the threat or action of suicide. Family members may feel rejected and accused. The weakness and alienation of a community is revealed. Everyone is left worse off. Suicide kills the individual, blights those close to the victim, frustrates the professional care system, and indicts the social environment that allowed it to occur. Thus, the psychological and moral consequences of suicide are just as important a concern as its lethal nature.

Aging and Suicide

We are instinctively appalled at the high rate of suicide among elderly white males and wonder what we are doing to and can do for this group. White males over the age of 75 have a suicide rate over seven times that in white females of the same age, and higher than the rate in any other age group. Cross-section data on the U.S. white population for 1963–66 show that in males, rates (per 100,000) rise from under 10 at age 15–24 to about 50 for those 75 years and older; in females the rates rise from about 3 to almost 11 at age 55–64 but level again to under 7 after age 75 (Atchley, 1980).

We may conjecture that, were care resources equal to those now devoted to cancer or the cardiovascular disorders

---

Barry J. Gurland is Director, Center for Geriatrics and Gerontology, Columbia University. Peter S. Cross is a Research Scientist.

to be directed at the social factors and individual vulnerabilities that precede suicide, the number of lives saved might rival that obtained in the more common cause of death.

The high suicide rates associated with advanced age have called our attention to many of the allegedly undesirable features of aging. Erikson (1950) regarded it as reflecting the despair of realizing that life had ceased to be meaningful and that it was too late to take an alternative pathway to integrity. Cameron (1972) showed that people of all ages felt that suicide was less objectionable in old than younger ages; not only conveying this feeling to the would-be suicide but also sometimes aiding and abetting the act. Others have pointed to the succession of losses that beset the elderly: losses of earnings, significant others, health, status, attractiveness, and other valued attributes.

Attempts of suicides are more likely to be successful in the elderly than in the young and the use of violent and certain means of suicide, e.g., gunshot and hanging as opposed to poisoning, is more common in the elderly than in the young; however, before one makes too much of this age variation in suicide, it is well to separate age from cohort effects. This point is made clearer by examining the suicide rates over a lifetime in a given generation (birth cohort) of persons. In such longitudinal data, the suicide rate of elderly white males does not regularly increase after the age of 60. Succeeding generations of elderly do have lower suicide rates giving the impression in cross-section data, of lower suicide rates in younger age groups. Thus, we need to examine more closely the causes of suicide in old age; it is not a straightforward matter.

Mental Illness as a Risk Factor

Sainsbury (1963, 1968) concluded that most elderly suicides are mentally ill. Winokur and Tsuang (1975) in a follow-up of psychiatric patients over 30 to 40 years found that although 5% had committed suicide, none of the control group consisting of nonpsychiatric patients had done so. Robins et al. (1959) found 94% of the suicides studied were mentally ill, 68% with affective disorder or alcoholism. In a series of 30 elderly suicides, Barraclough (1971) found that

87% were mentally ill, 63% with affective disorder, and the remainder suffering from a depressive illness in conjunction with terminal physical illness, alcoholism, or organic brain syndrome.

Depression is more likely to lead to suicide in older than younger patients (Gardner et al., 1964). In most elderly suicides the depression has lasted less than a year (Barraclough, 1971; Robins et al., 1959). This short duration indicates the urgency of intervention to prevent this ultimate consequence of depression. Unfortunately, the elderly person's first depression may be his last. One in 6 of depressives succeed in committing suicide compared with 1 in 100 of the general population. The seriousness of purpose of the elderly suicide is further indicated by an analysis of suicide notes: more than half of those written by elderly persons indicate a strong wish to die while those written by younger persons are much more aggressive and ambivalent with less than a quarter expressing a strong wish to die (Farberow and Shneidman, 1957). Nevertheless, the majority of the depressions associated with suicide in the elderly appear to be treatable and remediable. It has been calculated (Barraclough, 1972) that the appropriate use of lithium to prevent depressive relapses might prevent 20% of suicides.

Physical Illness and Depression

Next in importance to depression as a factor in elderly suicides is the presence of physical illness. Sainsbury (1955) found this important in 35% of his cases. Barraclough (1971) confirmed this relationship in a comparison of autopsies of suicidal and accidental deaths in the elderly; some of these physical disorders were obvious terminal cases of cancer, but surprisingly, some of them had not been evident prior to death. The importance of physical illness also figures large in the suicide notes of the elderly. Furthermore, countries with a high rate of suicide in the elderly also have high rates of death from chronic disorders, especially of a progressive and painful nature (Atchley, 1980).

In our own studies of the elderly in New York and London (Gurland et al., in press) we have found a very high correlation (.45) between physical disability and depression in the elderly. We were somewhat surprised to discover on a follow-up interview one year later that these associated depressions cleared up more frequently than did primary depression, i.e, without physical illness (Wilder, 1980). This suggests that a valid approach to depression associated with physical illness is to expect that improvement in the depression will occur if one can tide the elderly person over the initial impact of their disability and if one can relieve or at least control the progress of the disability so as to facilitate adjustment.

Isolation and Vulnerability

With the advent of depression or physical disability, the elderly who are *isolated* become very vulnerable to suicide. Those living alone constitute about half the elderly suicides (an overrepresentation of twofold). Recent isolates, i.e., those persons who have suffered a recent forced separation through bereavement or through divorce, are particularly vulnerable. Conversely, preferential and lifelong isolates seem well adjusted to that state as long as they remain well. It would improve our targeting of vulnerable groups if we cease to regard isolation itself as damaging and look rather to the type of isolation and its attendant events as the danger signals.

Marshall (1978), examining changes in suicide rates of U.S. white males over the period of 1948–1972, showed that the general socioeconomic conditions prevailing in the nation coincide with fluctuations in the rate of suicide. Over this period suicide rates decreased steadily with increases in the proportion of aged males receiving an income, increases in the real dollar Social Security income of husband-wife families, and increases in the proportion of the labor force covered by Social Security. Although factors such as war and the cohesiveness of communities also affected suicide rates, they were not as influential as economic conditions.

Also on this large scale of analysis, Low et al. (1981) examined changes in suicide rates in England and Wales over the 100 years between 1876 and 1975, concluding that the availability of toxic gas affected the number of suicides as a whole. Unemployment and alcohol consumption also explained some of the changes in suicide rates, especially among males. Finally, the war years were marked by dramatic drops in the suicide rates, consistent with Durkheim's (1897) hypothesis that war increases the collective sense of belonging and hence diminishes the tendency to suicide.

This background information should provide us with an insight into the need for prevention of suicide in the elderly, the profile of the suicide-prone elderly person, and the most promising means of intervening. The need for prevention is already self-evident. We turn now to synthesizing the profile of the suicide-prone person.

Profile of the Suicide-Prone Individual

Previous suicide attempts (which increase the risk of later successes sevenfold) and expressions of suicidal intent are obvious indicators but since first attempts are frequently successful in the elderly and since appeals for psychological help are frequently inhibited, one cannot rely on these direct indicators. The major indirect indicator is clearly depression, especially those with insomnia, agitation, hypochondriasis, self-neglect, or evidence of impaired memory (Barraclough et al., 1974; Farberow and McEvoy, 1966). The situation is even more ominous in those living alone, in those with conflict at home, and in males.

Some of these predictive factors have pointed relevance to modes of intervention. Those with symptoms such as insomnia or previous attempts at suicide are a highly vulnerable subgroup. In addition, factors of social vulnerability, such as isolation or successive use of alcohol, heighten the vulnerability. Finally, medical factors such as the conjunction of physical illness and the acquisition of prescription drugs identify a prime risk group.

Treatment of Depression

Depression in the elderly is remediable, just as it is in younger subjects, and deserves the same repertoire of treatments that is available to younger patients (Gurland and Toner, 1981). With the relief of depression, the suicidal impulses usually recede. Although severe and refractory depressions are the most likely to produce suicide, a substantial proportion of suicides have had a depression which was not recognized as severe or dangerous or was considered not to warrant specialized treatment. Our studies of representative samples of the community elderly indicate that about 13% of those 65 years or older have a clinical level of depression and that this group of elderly are very high users of psychoactive and potentially dangerous drugs. Unfortunately, we found fewer such depressives were being treated by antidepressants in New York than in London (Gurland et al., in press).

Clinical Implications of Predictors of Suicide

We need to discuss the implications for intervention of some of these other predictors of suicides. Insomnia is a predictor, partly because patients with this symptom have ready access to hypnotics, mainly barbiturates. Although the insomnia is often long-standing, the patient has frequently had an hypnotic renewed or initiated by prescription in the period immediately preceding the suicide.

Contact with a potential source of psychological help is probably common in the prodrome to suicide. In an English study (Barraclough, 1971), 90% of suicides among the elderly had seen a primary care physician within 3 months (often within a week) of the suicide; yet only 8% were referred to a psychiatrist. The vast majority (80%) of these subjects were on a psychoactive drug, but only 20% were on antidepressants and then, often on an inadequate dosage. These outpatient contacts are particularly significant because 90% of suicides are not inpatients. The period after discharging from inpatient status is a particularly dangerous time.

Unfortunately, the lines of communication between the elderly patient and the physician are often tenuous. Murphy (1975) investigated 49 suicides who had seen a physician within 6 months of death and found that the majority (35) of the suicides had made their intentions clear but less than half (39%) of the physicians involved recognized this: about half (25) of the suicides had clear evidence of depression but only 38% of the physicians made this diagnosis; and 16 of the 32 suicides who had taken an overdose had obtained their lethal dose from a single prescription. Improved identification of depression and its timely referral might be dependent on family, voluntary, or nonmedical contacts who are properly informed about the symptoms that signal the need for referral and who are skilled in obtaining the appropriate professional contacts.

That living alone is a predictor of suicide in the depressed elderly (by a factor of six times) underlines the importance of providing a supportive network, formal or informal, for those at risk for suicide. Bagley (1972) found evidence in a study of 30 American states to support Durkheim's view that social integration reduced suicide rates. It is those who are single and have never had a close social group to turn to who are most in jeopardy. Where the elderly person at risk for suicide has a family or relatives, they should be co-opted into the therapeutic effort; they should be informed of the symptoms of a depressive relapse and asked to bring the patient in for adjustment of treatment. Where a family is not available, it may be possible to construct a surrogate from community or voluntary organizations.

The excess rate of suicide in males compared with females is uniform across most western countries and seems to be true from puberty onwards. In the elderly it has been suggested that men accept physical dependency less well than do women and resort to alcohol where women would seek support from doctors, clergy, or other members of the support system. In general, it has been stated that women are more adaptable than men and can thus better accept old age. Whatever the merits of these hypotheses, the implications for intervention are that one should not overlook the necessity to strengthen the coping capacity and aid the adjustment of the elderly person who is facing a multitude of changes in life.

Curiously the period of retirement does not appear to be one of the more seriously provocative events as far as suicide is concerned. There is no surge of suicide rates in men either before or after the usual age of retirement (Atchley, 1980). Forced relocation, bereavement, and the advent of disability are more likely to be traumatic life events in old age.

One should not look for too close a relationship between the predictors of suicide and the identification of the individual in need. Barraclough and Pallis (1975) are of the opinion that "because methods of clinical assessment are imperfect and life events unpredictable, the forecasting of future suicide is impossible and may always be so." Rather, the net may have to be cast wider to lower the risk of suicide in the many elderly who are depressed and despairing.

Suicide Equivalents

Pursuing this expansive note, the prevention of suicide in the elderly should be targeted not only at explicitly suicidal behavior but at other self-destructive actions. Certain behaviors may lead to self-destruction but cannot confidently be labelled as suicidal because of uncertainty regarding the motivation behind them. Such behaviors have been termed indirect self-destructive behaviors by Nelson and Farberow (1977). In the elderly in nursing homes, such behaviors might include refusing food, noncompliance with medication regimes, conflict with other patients, and self-neglect. Nelson and Farberow (1980) found in a study of 99 male nursing home patients that these behaviors were associated with suicide risk, dissatisfaction with life, recent losses, and low religious commitment. Subjects who had no hope of returning to their families showed the most evidence of these behaviors. It appears that in situations where elderly persons have little in the way of positive change to look forward to, and are disabled, dispossessed and isolated, they may give vent to their feelings of despair through potentially self-destructive behavior which is not easily classified as suicidal.

The Effectiveness of Intervention

Efforts at intervention to reduce rates of suicide among the elderly do have a base of knowledge upon which to build; however, it is not certain whether efforts to date have been as effective as they might be. We have to do even better than before.

Community psychiatry services do appear to increase the referral of depressed elderly for specialized care (Sainsbury, 1965) and possibly to reduce the rate of suicide among this group (Walk, 1967). However, it is well known that the elderly are underrepresented in community mental health centers, in outpatient psychiatric clinics, and in private psychiatric practice (Gurland and Cross, 1982).

The introduction of a lay crisis intervention service for troubled people may reduce rates of suicide in younger subjects, but, at least as tested in England, the elderly tend not to know about or use such services (Atkinson, 1970). There is a need to ensure that services are known by the elderly and accessible physically and financially to them.

Furthermore, although a study by Bagley (1968) showed that in 15 cities with lay crisis intervention Samaritan services the suicide rates fell, whole in another 15 cities without such services the suicide rates rose. Barraclough (1972) replicated this study on a larger scale and was unable to find differences suggesting a therapeutic effect for Samaritan services. Lester (1974) similarly could not show an impact on suicide rates of suicide prevention centers in cities in the United States. Bridge et al. (1977) found only a minimal effect for suicide prevention centers in North Carolina. Studies on individual centers have not provided clearcut results either. Clearly the challenge of finding and adequately treating the depressed and suicidal elderly has not yet been vigorously enough addressed.

Brown (1979) accepts that suicide rates declined in Britain in the 1960s but doubts that this had much to do with the benefits of community psychiatry or the growth of Samaritan services. He points out that although mortality from suicide has decreased, suicidal behavior has probably increased. He attributes the reduced death rate from suicidal behavior to the saving of life due to improvements in ambulance and rescue services and to better hospital treatment of poisonings, to the replacement of barbiturates by the safer benzodiazepines, and to the lowering of the carbon monoxide content of domestic gas supplies. We need to do more toward reducing the availability and lethality of common means of suicide and toward improving our care of the actively suicidal person.

Welu (1977), noting that two thirds of suicide attempters receive no follow-up attention, established a community mental health center team to contact suicide attempters immediately after discharge from the emergency clinic. The team maintained continuity of treatment using an eclectic approach. A significant reduction of suicide reattempts and of alcohol or drug misuse was achieved compared with a control group.

What Can Be Done?

More and better training is essential. The training of primary care workers of all disciplines, whether medical, psychiatric, nursing, social work, or other front-liners, in the recognition of depression in the elderly and in appropriate treatment or referral is crucial. A suggestion has even been made that coroners (medical examiners) should inform health-care workers what has happened to their patients so that they might learn for the future (Barraclough, 1971).

Regarding services, we need to look at our successes and to be inspired by them. Something might be working. White male suicide rates appear to have been steadily falling among the elderly. Furthermore, the suicide rates in the United States are much lower than in some other countries, for example, in Hungary where rates are four times higher for elderly males than they are here (Atchley, 1980). It may well be that the broad front of social, economic, and medical programs for the elderly are as effective in reducing rates of suicide as are specific programs of suicide prevention. This seems like a good argument for continuing a broad front of efforts on behalf of the elderly while simultaneously attempting to improve the specificity of measures for primary and secondary suicide prevention.

Maintaining the current level of services as the population of elderly doubles in the next 40 years, will require our expanding twice the present effort or achieving twice the present efficiency. Careful planning and management of limited health and social resources will be essential. A massive educational effort must be undertaken. What can be projected for the future with respect to suicide rates in the elderly would seem to depend less on the changing demography than on what we and our policymakers do toward improving the quality of life and of health services for the elderly.

Epilogue

Dr. Bennett makes several points worthy of repeating:

1. Social isolation is not a singular entity but rather a phenomenon that, when it occurs in the elderly, must be evaluated in terms of past history and patterns.
2. Many isolates have prior histories of mental illness, and these persons can best be handled in long-term care facilities which have psychiatric support services available.
3. Many lifelong social isolates end up in institutions; however, there are significant numbers of these people residing in the community as well.

Dr. Gurland further elaborates on this subject by citing sudden involuntary isolation (whether created by bereavement or divorce) as a risk factor for suicide in the elderly and cautions that it is not isolation per se but rather the forced nature of this isolation.

Dr. Gurland discussed suicide as a problem with multivariate determinants, including mental illness, especially depressive disorder; physical disability; chronic illness and pain; and diminished social supports. He suggests that a broadened approach to improving the quality of life for the elderly through a range of programs and services would be preferable to a targeted suicide prevention program for the elderly; however, he cautions that it is very often not easy to overlook suicidal potential in elderly persons.

1. Learn to recognize mental illness in the older person. Depression is not a normal state.
2. Remember that physical illness may figure strongly in suicidal behavior and that behavioral adjustment can be facilitated by control of the progress of the disability. Optimize physical health and nutrition. Discuss the

patient's anxieties and inform him/her about illness. Alleviate pain as far as possible.
3. Target additions to those who are recent involuntary isolates, recently discharged from hospitalization for depression, or are resorting to alcohol to relieve depression; these groups are particularly vulnerable. Take failed suicide attempts seriously; in the elderly there is a high probability of a later successful suicide act.
4. Be alert to the most dangerous symptoms of depression such as insomnia, hypochondriasis, appetite changes, agitation, and self-neglect. Probe for feelings of despair and suicidal intent as appropriate. Consider hospitalization if depression is rapidly progressive, resistant to treatment, or accompanied by suicidal intent.
5. Keep in mind that depression in the elderly is treatable. However, to be effective, treatment must be vigorous, persistent, and carefully monitored; inadequate treatment can aggravate the condition. Relapse can also be minimized by continuing treatment.
6. Overcome common prejudices about the use of physical treatments such as medication or electro-shock. When properly and conservatively used, these treatments can be lifesaving. They are additional and not alternative to psychosocial treatments. Use the least toxic drug and limit hoarding of medications. Tide the patient over the long interval before treatment takes effect.
7. Encourage a broad-based system of informal supports. This can be helpful in promoting recovery, obtaining compliance with treatment, and improving reporting of danger signals. Social supports are even more crucial in those who live alone. The formal service system can also provide emotional support but must be readily accessible.
8. Relieve concrete social problems such as financial hardship and housing difficulties. Involve the patients in these solutions so as to increase their sense of mastery.
9. Be aware of ambulance and rescue services in the neighborhood.

Part IV

THEORETICAL AND PRACTICAL CONSIDERATIONS IN DEALING WITH THE HARD-TO-MANAGE

Prologue

The chapter contains three conceptual pieces. Monsignor Charles Fahey discusses the policy and ethical considerations involved in attempting to serve impaired elderly persons in the face of their resistances. Dr. Marcella Weiner reflects on working with these groups of impaired elderly from a psychoanalytic perspective. Rochelle Lipkowitz bridges the gap between the conceptual and the pragmatic, presenting an overview of general resistances to services by the elderly and by the professionals who serve them as well as specific issues in dealing with the hard-to-manage in crisis situations.

Policy and Ethical Concerns Regarding Interventions with the Acting-Out Elderly

Monsignor Charles Fahey

The subject of this publication is particularly timely as the nation debates the future of long-term care in the face of an ever-increasing older and more frail population. Economic considerations have led to the containment of acute care hospital beds, reduction in lengths of stay for those utilizing existing hospital beds, and a closer scrutiny of nursing home care. Psychotropic drugs, the theory of "normalization," and fiscal considerations have led states to a policy of deinstitutionalization or, more accurately, the diversion of patients from the state mental hospitals to various settings in the community. Nursing homes, health care, and community social agencies have become residual service systems in our communities. They have changed radically over the past 20 years. Despite a growth of one million new nursing home beds over the past 10 years, supply has not kept pace with the demand. While some limited supportive services are available for frail and vulnerable people in the community, the number of those whose behavior ranges from eccentric to the irrational has grown, troubling local communities and legislators alike.

Our primary concern is not the society that is disturbed by the bizarre behavior of marginal people but rather for these persons themselves. Our concern is that people be enabled to make choices and that they simultaneously be protected from making choices which are harmful to others as well as to themselves. Our concern is not only for those who are acting out but also for those who demonstrate a dimin-

---

Monsignor Charles Fahey is Director, Fordham University Gerontology Center.

ished capability for making choices and for seeking assistance. We are deeply concerned about the appropriateness of intervention in the lives of those who do not have the capacity to act for themselves.

The instinct of those in the helping professions is to follow a general civil liberties approach which stresses the autonomy and freedom of individuals. Yet, even as we champion this concept, we are increasingly aware of the hurts of those whose behavior is outside the established social norms and of the rights of society.

We have seen the plights of the persons of Love Canal among whom was an elderly gentleman who refused to leave. We saw interviews with the "old man of the mountain" who refused to leave his home at Mt. St. Helen and who is presumed to have been killed. We in New York are well accustomed to the "bag ladies" who make their home on the streets or in public places such as subway stations. I was recently called upon to be a consultant for a Jewish federation in a large metropolitan area (not New York) which was faced with a dilemma. Residents of a 202 Senior Citizen Housing project (202 Housing refers to a government-supported unit for the well elderly) and professionals of the federation had quite differing views regarding the frail tenants of that housing unit. The tenant council of the 202 project had petitioned the sponsoring group to evict certain members of their community who had become debilitated. The disability of some tenants was so severe and so constant as to require substantial professional intervention and thus allegedly contributed to a change in the character of the independent housing. The behavior of some persons was regarded as unacceptable. On the other hand, professionals of the family service agency serving the unit felt that a variety of social and medical services should be provided to persons in their own homes. They felt that if services were promptly and appropriately provided, premature institutionalization could be avoided and those disabled tenants would be able to remain in their home.

The Karen Quinlan and the Brother Fox cases both occurred in our immediate area and raised issues regarding the relationship of professional intervention and the courts.

English law, the basis of our American jurisprudence, has

judicial procedures to establish a person to act as a surrogate for a disabled person, in regard to his property and sometimes even his personal choices. It must be noted that the court's fundamental underlying approach is to assure that the best interests of a client are protected. The court itself does not become the decision maker for the disabled person. Rather, it designates a surrogate decision maker whose responsibility it is to assure the best interests of the client. This surrogate is expected to act as the client would have acted in a given circumstance, in accord with his or her values.

Concern for civil liberties, coupled with unfortunate discrimination and exploitation in many parts of American society, have led to a series of civil rights laws and due process procedures. However, law is sometimes a crass and gross tool. Constitutional and legal commentators are unanimous in noting that democracy depends upon socially responsible behavior of individuals. Law is a pedagogue, law directs, law constrains, but law is never able to reach into the most intimate of relationships of human beings and to deal with every case. Law is blind, and law can be severe and oppressive. There is a dictum of which we must be mindful: "difficult cases make bad law."

There are familiar instances in which law has been utilized to deal with individual problems only to find that there are unintended consequences of this approach which generate even greater problems.

General social questions have been addressed by an appeal to the courts, particularly where legislatures have been slow to act. *Brown v. Board of Education,* which outlawed separate but equal schools, is a celebrated example. In a more recent case, the Appellate Division of the Supreme Court of New York has developed procedures in the Brother Fox case, despite the fact that the issue had become moot by the reason of the death of Brother Fox. This decision is under appeal.

There are some indications, however, that judicial restraint is growing. The celebrated Willowbrook consent decree was occasioned by the State of New York's stipulation of a series of reforms regarding the care of those persons institutionalized at Willowbrook. A special panel was set up to monitor the ongoing operation of the institution. Subsequent action on the part of the State legislature not to fund this Willowbrook panel was appealed to a federal circuit court. In a recent decision, the court indicated that social policy should be determined by the State legislature rather than by the federal courts.

In an analogous case (Partham JR 99 s.c.p. 2493, 2496 (1979)), a majority of the Supreme Court agreed that voluntary institutionalization of a child by his/her parents need not be monitored by a court within the context of an adversary proceeding but rather could be monitored by a disinterested professional party.

While successful utilization of the judicial process to advance certain social causes gives rise to the temptation to use it in all difficult situations, it should be noted that the judicial process is at its best in adjudicating factual instances and dealing with past events in the context of the case. The court has no expertise in future behavior, particularly in noncriminal matters. The court is best in assuring due process, not in actually making a determination as to the best course of action to be taken.

I have discussed the court's role at some length in order to encourage professionals to exercise their proper responsibilities. We must act in an aggressive manner to intervene for those people who need our assistance. Our commitment to civil liberties, our concern about due process, and our concern about pluralism in society should not paralyze us in our efforts to act in a professional manner with our clients. The appropriateness of our activity as individuals and as agencies is governed not only by our framework of civil law but also by our ethical perspectives.

Each of us, implicitly or explicitly, acts ethically; that is, we have established values which influence our behavior. That which governs the interaction of the professional with the client is not licensure or regulation but rather the implicit contractual arrangement based upon the ethics of the particular profession. A patient goes to a doctor fully confident that a doctor's ethical stance is one which dictates that the client is assisted in being restored to health according to the dictates of the Hippocratic oath. By the same token, institutions or agencies which exist to help have ethics which dictate the behavior of those who work for them.

The word "profession" is borrowed from the religious life. When men and women enter the religious life, with the intent of taking vows of poverty, chastity, and obedience to serve God and neighbor, they enter a period of training, one of reflection and self-discipline. After this period they come before their peers and the whole community to profess their commitment. The helping disciplines in our culture have borrowed from this process of "professionalization." They, too, have a raison d'être, providing assistance to others within a definite set of values. A person entering such a profession develops not only knowledge and skills but also learns to exercise certain prescribed values, i.e., an ethic.

There is a need for service programs to identify those values or that ethical stance within which their services are rendered. A group of people working together for others might be characterized as a community and as moral persons. As an individual is sick or healthy, wise or foolish, efficient or inefficient, emotionally mature or immature, so, too, is a group. And as a person develops values which influence his or her behavior, so, too, does a group. Individuals and groups must take a systematic approach to behavioral values, and this we call the ethic which guides their work. A characteristic of those who act ethically is their struggle to identify the basic values in their lives. It is something that goes on continually. I do not propose to give you a ready-made set of values, but invite you instead to enter as an individual and agency into a process of reflection on the ethics of our work as service providers.

Among those values which are likely to evolve from such a process of reflection are a commitment to the dignity of people, a healthy respect for the individual and his uniqueness, a desire to maximize a person's functional capabilities, a desire to work collaboratively on a continuing basis with a person who is frail and vulnerable, a commitment to bear appropriate responsibility for the overall well-being of a person, a commitment to confidentiality, a commitment to deal with a person honestly, and a commitment to act on behalf of a person with diminished capabilities, in accordance with that person's values, history, and life-style.

Even as we consider our own behavior and the behavior of those groups of which we are part, it is sound to examine the question of social expectations. As we consider the formal intervention of persons in the lives of others, we should also consider the control of a person's behavior by those who live in the same community. Groups have a right and even a responsibility to identify those behaviors which are acceptable or unacceptable for individuals who wish to be part of that group. The smaller and more intimate a group, the more likely the group will have a significant impact on the lives of its members. Families have the right to establish rules and norms for family members. Residential facilities should have rules for social behavior if persons are to function within the context of that particular setting. Senior citizen centers, hospitals, adult homes, and nursing homes have every right and, in fact, a responsibility to establish social norms, so that those utilizing their services know what behavior is expected of them.

As long as the rules are reasonable, are applied fairly and equitably, and can be justified, it is entirely appropriate, both from an ethical and legal point of view, for them to exist. To expect persons to live within the context of such rules or else to accept the consequences of disregarding them is entirely proper. Many would argue that these social constraints are necessary if individuals are to act with freedom and realize the fullness of their personalities.

The subject of the acting-out elderly is a challenge indeed. It is most appropriate for us to reflect together on the frailty and vulnerability in which we all share, so that we may consider humbly and honestly the ways in which we can most effectively and ethically intervene in the lives of others—*both* for their benefit and ours as well.

Reflections on the Hard-to-Manage Elderly

Marcella Bakur Weiner, EdD

The hard-to-manage elderly are often said to be "acting out." Perhaps a better description of this group would be "acting in." For the formal properties of "acting-out" read as follows:

> The partial discharge of instinctual tension that is achieved by responding to the present situation as if it were the situation that originally gave rise to the instinctual demand . . . . It is an acting which unconsciously relieves inner tension and brings a partial discharge to warded-off impulses . . . . The present situation . . . is used as an occasion for the discharge of repressed energies. (Hinsie and Campbell, 1960)

The individual thus "acts in"—this being conceived of as an habitual pattern, developed over a life span and considered or felt by that person to be the only response to a typically frustrating situation. The resultant behavior, often of great annoyance and distress to others and even to the person himself, is the result of a long-term conflict between his own impulses over which he lacks control and the frustrating external world. He thus "acts in," in accordance with patterns developed over many years of living; congruent with a personality structure he has owned for 60, 70, 80 or more years; and in harmony with a message he is trying to relate to the outer world, no matter how bizarre, unacceptable, or deviant the behavior coating that message may appear to those around him.

Marcella Bakur Weiner is Adjunct Professor of Psychiatry, Brooklyn College (CUNY).

The older adult, whether labeled "senile" or not, is a decidedly unique individual. That fact seems simplistic, yet is overlooked by many as we attempt to understand and help the person whose behavior has been his unique style of relating to the world for over half a century and more—a behavior which had its origins in the very early years and which has continued in its complexity over a lifetime.

Perhaps it would be helpful to examine why it is that helping professionals often exhibit an avoidance response when dealing with a group of older adults labeled "senile," "acting-out," "deviant," etc. If we were to consider situations we tend to avoid, possibly those which render us helpless would be first on the list. A feeling of helplessness is the flip side of that much-desired feeling, mastery. Feeling masterful in situations gives us a sense of competence, self-esteem, and worth, which do so much for the continuance of a positive self-image. This feeling of mastery is reciprocal in nature in that, felt inside by us as a positive emotional response to the world, we can then, in turn, act upon that world in a positive way. Thus, the inner experience and the outer environment reinforce each other, to the benefit and continuance of both. The opposite may occur in situations where feelings of helplessness are engendered. We are left, bereft of our self-esteem, in wonderment at our felt lack of competence, and with discomfort, almost of a physical nature, gnawing at our insides. It is no wonder that a typical response, similar to that of animals being shocked, is to "flee the scene." Like our patients (clients), we, too, are "acting in"—in accordance with an impulse which is to feel that which is noxious or intolerable, a facet of the human need to survive.

Nonacceptance of disruptive behavior is not the same as nonunderstanding. Understanding is more than a passive acceptance of intolerable behaviors; rather, more in keeping with the natural curiosity drive intrinsic to all healthy persons, it is active in its nature, intentional rather than random, and has as its goal the defining of behaviors in a systematic fashion so that a continuous pattern can emerge for scrutiny, and the ultimate goal of treatment accomplished.

That so-called "senile" person, however desocialized and for whatever reasons, has *chosen* (emphasis mine), consciously and unconsciously, a way of responding to the world which best explains him. That is, of the multitude of behaviors, actions, thoughts, feelings, ideas he can exhibit, some choice was made. This choice was/is unique to him and only to him and is the consequence of a particular way of relating to himself and others, exhibited over many, many years. This style, this stamp, needs to be observed and respected, for then and only then can we, the helping persons in his environment, have a clue to what the real message is. And it is only then that we can close the gap—the gap between our world and his. Within our working space, we can share the patient's world, and without condemnation, moral evaluation, and pejorative labeling. In traditional psychotherapy, this is often referred to as the "therapeutic alliance," and certainly it is therapeutic (of benefit to others) to have an alliance with the world of persons we wish to help. Similarly, more recent theory has discussed the therapeutic stance of "empathic attunement" (Mahler). That view holds that we interpret the patient's world as it appears to him rather than as we see it or as we wish it to be. Once this is accomplished, this theory holds, the patient/client's ego functions will improve along with the basic factor held critical to all good functioning—one's own self-esteem.

As a therapist, I believe that not only must we deliver a response which is realistic and expected from us to confirm the patient's "real" (observable and consensually validated) world, we need also understand what he is trying to say through "unacceptable" behaviors. Neither is mutually exclusive. For while we deliver our response, our scientific minds, always ready to collect and interpret data, can gather clues from the patient's behavior as to the meaning of these behaviors. Our response should then include both an understanding of the manifest and the latent content since both are part of the same person. Both also talk to the behavior as an act and the feeling underlying that behavior. Again, ideas and feelings are part of a unit and need not be separated. Most importantly, once this position is assumed and we professionals interpret the patient's true intent, he feels "understood"—that feeling being related to all examples of "cure" (Paul, 1963).

We also need to understand and appreciate that behaviors considered "good" in the outside world may not be effective in a facility housing the aged. The particular trait factor found to be associated with successful institutional adaptation . . . loaded highly on activity, aggression, and narcissistic body image, according to Turner, Tobin and Lieberman (1972). Furthermore, this cluster of traits

> suggests that a vigorous, if not combatative style is facilitory for adaptation. The personality style . . . most apt to survive in a facility is one of being intrusive, of actively seeking interaction, of aggressively relating, and of insisting on responsivity from others regarding physical attentiveness. (Turner, Tobin, and Lieberman, 1972)

They suggest, in their summary, that the traits are reflective of a style which is "narcissistic in its orientation as well as hostile and controlling." Thus, for the older adult placed in a facility such as a nursing home or adult home, preinstitutional personality traits need to exist which are congruent with the demands of that new environment. It may be that the older adult considered "difficult" at best and "acting-out" or "impossible" at worst may do astonishingly well in an institutional environment such as a nursing home. Provocative as this may be, further research is needed to define this concept more clearly.

Most pertinent to our discussion of the difficult-to-manage elderly are Ruth Bennett's ongoing research and pioneer efforts in the field of social isolation. She makes the very cogent point that critical periods need to be established for social isolation, recognizing that isolation prior to entry into a facility for the aged was most related to poor adjustment immediately after entry. Her contributions regarding the marked distinctions between involuntary and voluntary isolates have long been noted. It would seem that the voluntary isolate with the poorest adjustment and who is most difficult to approach to the dismay of dedicated staff, can be defined as the "loner" who, as Dr. Bennett so accurately states, has no doubt had this life-style for an interminable time. Were we to peel away the top layers of this defensive structure, it might be possible to gain some understanding of what, in the original situation, years and years ago, possibly in early childhood, was so threatening so that the only way to survive was withdrawal from human contact. For that is what the voluntary isolate has done; again, adaptively from the point of view of the need to survive, he had withdrawn in order to protect himself, as does the child from the hot stove.

Interaction with others, a mutual give-and-take so familiar to us in our everyday world, is interpreted by him as a threat to survival. He therefore holds tenaciously to the only form of "self-soothing" (Kohut, 1977) he knows, i.e., that of pulling into himself and shutting out the rest of the world. Observing him 50, 60, or 70 years after this behavior became a part of his personality structure, it is hard for us to imagine him as a young child convinced that the only way to survive is to learn not to trust anyone except himself. The world, seen from his young eyes, must have appeared cold, aloof, unavailable, and, at worst, potentially intent upon destroying him. Defensive behavior always involves perceived threat; and so it is with our "voluntary isolate." Once on this road, perhaps lonely to us but necessary to him, the reading of social cues ceases, and in old age, he is a babe in the woods seeing all trees as alike, if indeed he recognizes them at all. His only world is his inner world and his only comfort comes from his experience within himself, hollow as it may be since the imprints of images of long ago—parents and others—are negated in an attempt to wipe out that which was not intolerable.

How then do we help them? Perhaps one hopeful note is found in Dr. Bennett's statement that "isolates were found to be highly persuasible." This would suggest that even within the term "social isolates of a voluntary nature" there are gradations or levels of isolation. These gradations, from the standpoint of developmental theory seem to have arisen from the degree of severity of trauma in early life. Simply, the person who suffered the least from an environment seen as threatening has more potential for change than one whose trauma was severe. The basic problem is how to discover the degree of trauma in a person now 70 or 80 years old when little or no data are available. As social scientists, we need to work with data, for only the uncovering of evidence can lend credence to tentative hypotheses about human behavior. Yet, contrary to working with children, younger people or unimpaired older adults who have recall, working with frail older persons often prevents our accumulating data from the best source—the older adult himself. How do we solve this dilemma? The only possibility, it seems, is to develop our sensitivities and our observational abilities. That is, even when the category of "voluntary isolate" is assigned to the older person, that categorization, as helpful as it may be, perhaps could be further refined. Psychologically, it would mean attempting to understand the world as that person defines it through his behaviors, in this case, little or no interaction with others. Careful scrutiny could then establish limits as to what approaches might or might not be useful to that person and what types of environments could be most conducive to positive interactions, no matter how limited.

To conclude, the "acting-out" elderly are perceived as difficult to manage. Understandably, we, in our helplessness and frustrated attempts at treatment, often ignore this population, preferring to work with others who offer us more immediate gratification and affirmation of our effectiveness as mental health practitioners. Yet, if we were to accept and understand the behaviors symptomatic of that constellation termed "acting-out," recognizing that there is a message, a theme, being played out, the rewards for both our patients and ourselves could be great.

"Forcing" Services: What Can You Do for the Unwilling Client?

Rochelle Lipkowitz, RN, MS

The concept of "forcing" services which connotes doing for, rather than collaborating with, clients has onerous implications in an era characterized by consumerism. This is especially so when the clients are elderly, a group which is often seen as especially vulnerable and subject to abuse. In addition to the negative public image cast by such forcing, it also poses a clinical dilemma, for inducing dependency and/or helplessness can be a negative outcome in work with older people. It is because of extraordinary resistances to both the provision and the receipt of necessary services that techniques have evolved among health professionals, who have grown concerned about the lack of appropriate care for the elderly. Yet, forcing services on unwilling clients may not be the only means by which required care can be administered. In many cases, it may be possible to accomplish the same ends by identifying specific resistances to care—whether these resistances emanate from the client or from society—and dealing with them. However, in some cases, the resistances to care emanate from the very impaired elderly who are frequently so ill that without immediate care their lives are in jeopardy. For them, there is no time to interpret and deal with resistances. Services must be forced upon them. Yet these people are often considered least attractive and are neglected by members of the helping professions who do not know how to deal with them.

In addition, it is important to attend to a warning that is implicit in the forcing of services. One cannot always know

---

Rochelle Lipkowitz is Research Nurse Specialist, Resnick Gerontology Center, Albert Einstein College of Medicine.

if forcing services to ameliorate immediate danger may expose clients to later danger of an even greater magnitude which may ultimately shorten life, i.e., individuals may be placed after a fire or a crime in a "better" milieu to which they may not adapt. Thus the relocation may actually cause them to become more impaired.

In this paper, the various types of resistances to care which may be encountered when dealing with elderly clients will be described, as well as suggestions for intervention. Specific techniques of "forcing" services in life-threatening situations will also be described.

Techniques of Recognizing and Dealing with Resistances to Care-Ageism

The attitudes of many who are responsible for the health care of the elderly are often affected by "ageism," a term coined by Butler (1977) to describe the prejudices and stereotypes applied to older people purely on the basis of their age. Comfort (1976) has pointed out these prejudices are part of the psychic make-up of the elderly themselves, having been inculcated during their youth. As they age, they maintain these same beliefs and thus become part of the group practicing age discrimination. While in most groups, coping mechanisms are developed to deal with discriminatory behavior, the elderly, because of their beliefs, find themselves on both sides of the issue. They hold the same stereotypes which they cannot accept in others. Many feel that being debilitated or ill is their "lot in life" and, therefore, do not seek help for what they believe is inevitable. Senility and a host of other medical problems are thus accepted as part of "normal" aging. "What do you expect, you're getting old" is a common response from doctors, nurses, and other health professionals and reinforces their own negative attitudes. And, of course, the acceptance by elderly clients serves to reinforce the therapeutic nihilism of the professionals.

Fear and Shame

Fear or shame can inhibit the elderly from reaching out for required care. The problem of stigmatization applies to more than the need for psychosocial assistance. Earlier patterns of distrust continue in the elderly and cause them to experience shame when requested to expose their needs to "outsiders." Furthermore, the physical disfigurement, which often accompanies arthritic type illnesses, or the sense of loss of physical beauty in those who see only youth as beautiful are sources of shame and consequently of avoidance of services. Additional avoidance responses can be seen in aged members of minority groups who withdraw from professionals who do not speak their language or who are unaware of ethnic customs.

Poverty

Many of the elderly live in deprivation to the degree that they lack food, drugs, or a telephone in the house. However, government programs for the elderly are still controversial and poorly implemented. Obviously if essential services were guaranteed to the elderly, being poor would be less threatening. The present requirements for special cards and special benefits require extensive paper work and involvement with a complex bureaucracy. The need for frantic hustling simply to survive is a problem the elderly cannot contend with. Thus, they intentionally avoid seeking services to avoid hassles.

Lack of Information and Availability of Services

Various agencies have information and referral services, and radio, television, and other news media play some role in relaying necessary information to the older population. Many older people do not take advantage of services to which they are entitled because they face difficulties in the simple process of enrolling for them because of the bureaucratic processes. Moreover, once enrolled, they may find that no appropriate services are available.

The Medical Approach

While most professionals recognize that the treatment of older people requires a comprehensive biopsychosocial approach, this appears to be honored more in theory than in fact. Butler and Lewis (1977) have noted that older people are not seen in proportion to their emotional and psychiatric needs as outpatients in psychiatric clinics, community mental health centers, or in the offices of private psychiatrists or nonmedical therapists. Only 2% of persons seen in psychiatric clinics are over 60 years of age, while only 4.5% of those seen in community mental health centers are over age 65. On the other hand, Kane (1981) found that these same elderly receive a disproportionate amount of medical diagnosis and treatment compared with younger patients. Thus a curious paradox exists.

This disparity in utilization is a reflection of two factors. On the one hand, medical professionals dealing with the elderly find it easier to concentrate on concrete presenting medical symptoms than to deal with the underlying psychological and social problems. This is confounded by the fact that elderly individuals share the same feeling of stigma associated with the need for psychosocial assistance as do other members of this society and, if left to act independently, make infrequent requests for such services. The concentration on concrete medical services has potentially disastrous consequences. One of these is iatrogenesis: Provision of inappropriate medical services without attention to underlying psychosocial and environmental factors may lead to deterioration in overall health status among the elderly rather than improvement. Rather than perpetuating these disparities it would be of great value to address the resistances directly both to the elderly themselves and to the client or to treating professionals.

Independence vs. Dependence

Many elderly refuse assistance because they feel it will destroy their independence and take away their individuality. They view various interventions that are offered to them as alien and part of an "establishment" in which they have no belief. These negative feelings may emanate from the elderly's view of professionals and institutions as self-serving, insensitive to the needs of older citizens, or wanting to change old life patterns. For whatever reason, necessary interventions can be attempted only if these various beliefs are recognized and a trustful relationship is established.

Psychiatric Problems

The common feeling of hopelessness about psychiatric problems often prevents individuals from seeking assistance with them. This is, of course, further exacerbated by inadequate Medicare coverage for psychiatric care. For example, Medicare places a limitation of $250.00 per year on outpatient psychiatric services, while no such limit is placed on medical care. While there are unlimited benefits for inpatient medical care under Medicare, there is a 180-day lifetime limit for psychiatric inpatient care. This has led to a general neglect of the psychiatric problems of the elderly. An especially difficult group are those older individuals with paranoid symptoms. When such individuals have accompanying medical problems, they become a serious cause for concern, for their very lives are threatened by their reluctance to place trust in any other person. Great patience and insight are required for working with such people. Enlisting family or friends can be helpful in dispelling paranoid fears. After trust has developed, individuals may avail themselves of medication and psychotherapy which can often alleviate symptoms.

Demented Patients and Their Families

Because of their poor memory and judgment, demented patients often have difficulty establishing trusting relationships. A sensitive and friendly worker is needed to overcome resistance from such a client because forcing services may bring out great hostility in such individuals. Home visits are particularly helpful, for in their own environment, these clients feel more comfortable and in control and are more apt to establish trust in a new person offering help. Families of senile people have difficulties in this area as well. It is hard to accept regressive and sometimes bizarre behavior and to recognize the need for round-the-clock assistance. Because these difficulties continue over an extended period of time, often with inadequate support services for the family, many family caretakers develop ambivalence and unconsciously, simultaneously love and hate the afflicted person for whom they are responsible. It is difficult for them to handle their own increasing rage and lack of gratification, and guilt becomes a prevalent emotion. When this occurs, it is common to see such family members overcompensate by assuming total responsibility for the care of the senile person and resisting any offers of outside assistance. If both they and the senile clients are to be adequately served, such family members cannot simply be accepted as responsible adults. They have organized their days around assuming this caretaker role and have essentially "no other life." These family members must be recognized as patients in their own right who, as a result of their own emotional conflicts, refuse needed service. At such times it may become necessary for a responsible professional to counsel such family members and address the symptoms of guilt which prevent the client and the caretaker from accepting care.

Techniques of Forcing Services

It must be remembered that the phrase "forcing services" is actually a reference to infringement on individual civil rights. For this reason, any professional who decides to move in this direction must be extremely cognizant of the local laws, since civil rights are among the most cherished in our society and are therefore very carefully legally protected. State laws vary in their specific approaches to the topic about to be addressed but most have similar provisions as those of New York State, which will be used as a model for discussion. Professionals are urged to consult their own legal agencies before proceeding with any form of forcing services.

In general, the major reason for forcing services on an adult is a finding that he/she is so mentally impaired as to be unable to care for him/herself suitably. This applies even to the provision of lifesaving medical treatments, regardless of the severity of illness, unless the patient has first been declared legally incompetent. Obviously, in a situation in which mental illness has so impaired an individual that he is considered to be in a life-threatening situation, hospitalization is required. Every state has a mental hygiene law which prescribes the situations and techniques to be used in such circumstances.

In New York State, the Mental Health Law describes two forms of admission to psychiatric hospitals which can be utilized for objecting patients.

Emergency Admission

The first is the *emergency admission for immediate observation, care, and treatment*. Only a specified group of hospitals has been given the right to admit patients under this section of the law. Therefore, before proceeding with such a hospitalization, it is wise to check to see whether the intended hospital has such legal right. This particular form of admission is to be used only for patients "alleged to have a mental illness for which immediate observation, care, and treatment in a hospital is appropriate, and which is likely to result in serious harm to himself or others." The latter phrase is described specifically as:

> (1) substantial risk of physical harm to himself as manifested by threats of or attempts at suicide or serious bodily harm or other conduct demonstrating that he is dangerous to himself, or (2) substantial risk of physical harm to other persons as manifested by homicidal or other violent behavior by which others are placed in reasonable fear of serious physical harm.

Involuntary Admission

Such conditions do not cover all of the circumstances in which an acting-out elderly person might be felt to be in need of hospitalization. Therefore, the mental health law provides another avenue for such admission, which is the *involuntary admission on medical certification*. This form of admission can be forced upon an individual if, in the written opinion of two examining physicians (ordinarily psychiatrists) who have each examined the patient within 10 days of hospitalization, the person

> has a mental illness for which care and treatment as a patient in a hospital is essential to such a person's welfare and whose judgment is so impaired that he is un-

able to understand the need for such care and treatment.

Before such certification can be performed, a request, in the form of a petition must be executed by an individual who either resides with the patient, the nearest relative or committee of the patient, an officer of a home in which the patient resides, or the director of community services or social services. It is apparent that this is a complicated means of arranging for a hospitalization, but in most cases it is a better technique than the emergency admission section, for it requires the agreement of someone rather than the mental health professional who decides that admission is required.

In the event that the elderly individual resides alone, it may be necessary to utilize the emergency admission section. In theory it is not difficult for the professional who is working with the individual, or a psychiatrist at the hospital to which the patient is brought to consider the behavior exhibited as posing a serious danger to the person's life. Such behavior could emanate from the variety of disorders affecting the mentation of elderly individuals. In a recent evaluation of 100 outpatients brought to a geriatric clinic with complaints of organic mental disorder, 59% were diagnosed as primary degenerative dementia, 14% as multi-infarct dementia, 10% as dementia associated with alcoholism, 8% as dementia associated with specific neurologic disease, 3% as delirium, 24% as depression, and 3% as schizophrenia (Maletta et al., 1982). Unfortunately, with the possible exception of delirium, overt suicide threats in the presence of depression, or a floridly psychotic schizophrenic state, the majority of these conditions would not necessarily appear bizarre or unusual to a casual observer. This becomes important when it is necessary to utilize force to extract the individual from the home and bring him to a hospital. Ordinarily the police are called in such instances, but they, too, have become increasingly cautious regarding infringing on civil rights. Many precincts have been expressly ordered not to assist in removing individuals from their homes, unless the behavior appears overtly dangerous or threatening to the policemen. Therefore, it would be wise for the professional dealing with such situations to establish a relationship with the local police precinct to clarify the rules under which they operate and to indicate to them the nature of the professional services being offered. The police can be a valuable ally in this area only if the alliance is established before the difficulties occur.

Protective Services

There are times, however, when, in spite of the finest professional opinion, there appears to be no way to work within the restrictions of the Mental Health Law. At such times, it is wise to turn to an agency known as Protective Services for Adults, which is usually a division of the State Department of Social Services. This is a service mandated by federal regulations to provide services primarily to the impaired elderly, living alone and fearful of losing control of their lives. The organization is aware of the difficulties posed by the conflict between respect for civil rights, and the need for intervention when a potentially hazardous situation exists. When such a situation occurs, this agency can utilize its established legal protective services to:

> use legal authority and procedures on behalf of an individual who cannot manage his money, is exploited or is in danger; which involve court action to determine whether an older person is incapable of managing his own property or affairs; and which may result in the establishment of some form of trust relationship or commitment to an institution for such an individual.

It is unfortunate that this valuable agency is not widely known by professionals in the field. Since each state has its own regulations establishing the agency and the techniques by which it is contacted, it is recommended that all professionals or centers dealing with elderly clients make contact with their local Department of Social Service office and obtain information which will permit liaison with Protective Services for Adults.

In summary, forcing services on unwilling, acting-out elderly patients is a ticklish task, replete with complexities, both legal and clinical, and should be attempted only when a true emergency exists, and/or all other attempts at overcoming resistances have failed. It would be Pollyannish, however, to assume that such situations do not occur. When they do arise, it is often in an unanticipated situation, and at extremely inconvenient times. Therefore, it is wise for any professional or agency to prepare in advance in order to avoid last minute hysterics and helplessness.

What Can Be Done on a Practical Level?

1. *Recognize the resistances.* If the resistances which have been described are identified and attempts made at their elimination, a reduction in the amount of forced services would occur. A direct approach to elderly patients about the need for psychosocial intervention might alleviate some of the existing therapeutic nihilism. Likewise, physicians need to be apprised of the importance of psychosocial intervention for improvement of well-being.

2. *Improve communication* between and among health professionals and patient/clients. The development of a cooperative, consultative relationship among all health professionals, including physicians, could make them allies in persuading patients to seek and accept needed services.

3. *Education.* The resistances which are related to ageism are a societal problem which must be addressed by education on many levels. Fear and shame among the elderly themselves can best be dealt with by the development of group programs for older persons in which difficulties are openly discussed and in which feelings are shared among peers. This same psychosocial educational approach could benefit those caretakers who require support in handling their elders. Education of health professionals about aging as a developmental process as well as the disease aspects must be included in the various curricula.

4. *Increase availability of services and accessibility to them.* The resistance to treatment of the elderly which is related to the lack of availability of services is a social-political issue. The only approach to this is a political one.

5. *Advocacy.* Professionals dealing with elderly patients must become advocates for their clientele. They must take

affirmative action on behalf of the elderly, so that we as a society may become responsive to their needs in a more positive way. The aim is to develop a system in which all individuals are treated with respect and dignity. To avoid these difficult issues and to accept the easier approach of forcing services is to consign great numbers of our elderly citizens to a status somewhat less than human.

6. Learn the applicable sections of your state mental health law.

7. Establish liaison with a local psychiatric hospital, learn about its strengths and limitations, and learn of alternative hospitals which can provide missing services.

8. Establish liaison with the local police precinct so that they will be helpful in times of emergency.

9. Establish liaison with local Protective Services for Adults, that they may be contacted in specified situations.

Epilogue

This section, more than any other, provides a framework for the reasons why we as professionals find the mentally impaired elderly so hard to manage. There are some times when we may have cause to wonder who is doing the acting-out—they? we? society?

How can we respect a person's civil liberties while simultaneously protecting them from harming themselves or others? Who is to decide what is best in the presence of diminished capacity and the absence of a significant other? Where does the value of the law leave off?

Even where there are willing clients, adequate services may not be available. Given shrinking resources and an ever-increasing number of potentially needy elderly clients, how can we maximize those resources already in place? How can we integrate strategies that we know work, e.g., education, crisis intervention, family support, day care, team approach, respite care, protective services, etc.? And how can we get funding for these needed clients? We have more questions than answers at this point.

Part V

A PRAGMATIC APPROACH TO THE MENTALLY FRAIL ELDERLY

Prologue

In this section are some accounts of strategies that have been used in working with the acting-out elderly. Dr. Aronson discusses the family system and its actual and potential interactions with the health and social service systems and strategies that may be useful in maintaining or enhancing the role of the family in managing the hard-to-manage or acting-out elderly.

Ms. Weiner describes the experience of the Bronx Mobile Geriatric Crisis Team and its role in serving mentally frail elderly in their own homes.

Drs. Mesnikoff and Wilder describe the Community Support System program, a model for serving the mentally frail elderly in adult homes.

Mr. Pommerenck describes a specialized day care program and the related technique of attitude therapy.

The Case of the Bronx Mobile Geriatric Crisis Team

Sophie Weiner, MSW

The Geriatrics Committee of the Bronx Federation of the New York City Department of Mental Hygiene identified the major area of its concern as the delivery of comprehensive services to the frail elderly and identified that there was a glaring gap in service delivery capability in the borough of the Bronx. The committee was seeking the development of a capability for response to crisis by trained personnel within the mentally frail person's own environment. The committee applied for funds to establish a boroughwide crisis team which could pull together resources and a plan of treatment and thus often prevent hospitalization and/or nursing home placement by reaching the person before the crisis had reached the point that the person could no longer manage his/her resources or strengths. The Geriatrics Committee asked the Jewish Association for Services for the Aged (JASA) to become the sponsoring agency, and a crisis team was funded for a period of 3 years. A consortium of mental health providers was formed to ensure cooperation, to act as a liaison between and among agencies, and to serve as a supportive resource for the team.

The staff of the Mobile Geriatric Crisis Intervention Team was comprised of a psychiatrist (part-time), a social worker, coordinator, a psychiatric nurse, and a homemaker/housekeeper.

The team was charged, within its capacity to do so, to accept all requests for emergency home visits or visits to nonpsychiatric geriatric program sites such as senior citizens centers in any part of the borough of the Bronx, New York City, a borough with a very high proportion of elderly over 75.

The crisis team worked closely with the consortium agencies, the various mental health provider agencies in the Bronx, accepting referrals from them, intervening as appropriate, and referring clients back to them for ongoing follow-up after the initial crisis was resolved. After some initial problems, the team fulfilled its goals. It helped many clients to avoid hospitalization and/or nursing home placement. In a few instances, the timely intervention saved lives. The team was able to coordinate services for patients who had both medical and psychiatric problems. The team was especially effective because of the availability of backup by JASA which could provide concrete services, such as the transportation, relief funds, and/or additional homemaking services needed to fulfill a treatment plan.

The team approach provided an extended family for the client, and team members often interchanged roles. In some instances the clients shared confidences, not revealed to other team members, with the homemaker, who, in actuality, spent the most time with them.

I would like to share a case history with you:

> Ms. F. was referred to the crisis team by a local hospital. She was a 74-year-old, unmarried woman whose 95-year-old mother had just died at the hospital. Ms. F. lived with her mother most of her life and was extremely attached to her. The mother's death precipitated a crisis for Ms. F.; she became uncontrollable and had to be sedated while at the hospital. Afterwards, she made numerous suicidal references and the staff of the hospital, extremely concerned, referred her to the crisis team. There was no other family, and there were no other visible social supports. Because the situation was urgent, the team visited her right away. During the week of Shiva (Jewish mourning period), Ms. F. expressed a fear of sleeping in her apartment alone. The team provided homemaking help from relief funds for that week.
>
> The following week, the team visited Ms. F. for further follow-up. She was extremely depressed, crying off and on throughout the interview. She did talk some-

what about her conflicts and guilt triggered by her mother's death. The team tried to help her understand that her mother's illness had been so serious that death was inevitable, no matter what Ms. F's efforts had been. This explanation seemed to help Ms. F. somewhat, but the team psychiatrist felt that anti-depressant medication was indicated, and prescribed it at this visit.

The team's homemaker went to visit Ms. F. regularly, twice a week. She reinforced the worker's counseling efforts and urged Ms. F. to openly express her grief and loss, and also encouraged her to use the strengths she did have. Ms. F. was a great animal lover and gradually began to take on a nursing role to stray dogs. This arrangement was so beneficial to her that she was encouraged to volunteer some time to the A.S.P.C.A.

The team called Ms. F. frequently to check the intake of her medication, about which she was ambivalent and inconsistent. Eventually, the team nurse engaged Ms. F.'s local physician to encourage Ms. F. to take her medication. This local physician agreed to follow Ms. F. after the unit terminated with her.

As the team provided constancy and support through visits and telephone calls, Ms. F. gradually began to reintegrate herself back into living again. Ms. F. was encouraged toward greater autonomy, and began once again to participate in her informal social network. Teenagers came to her and walked her dogs, and she participated in a group at a local cafe. At the time of the homemaker's last visit before the case was closed, she noted that Ms. F. had a gentleman friend visiting her and otherwise appeared to be doing better. (Jupa, 1977)

In this case, the team was able to treat Ms. F.'s severe depression while maintaining her in the community. Psychiatric hospitalization was successfully avoided.

Unfortunately, despite the success of the crisis team, no replacement funding could be found upon termination of the initial 3-year funding. Though I am saddened by the termination of the Bronx Mobile Crisis Unit, I recommend that it be used as a model for a low-cost-effective intervention with frail elderly in the community and that other similar programs be funded. Whether they are funded through a social agency or through a psychiatric agency is probably irrelevant; the important aspects are flexibility, mobility, immediacy of response, and provision of concrete services as needed.

The Community Support System Programs: A Model for Serving the Mentally Frail in Adult Homes

Alvin Mesnikoff, MD
David Wilder, PhD

As was noted in Part II, the private proprietary home for adults (PPHA or adult home) has become a major community residential resource for the deinstitutionalized mentally ill. The history of these facilities is clouded by poor monitoring and numerous reports of poor conditions and inadequate care. There were some early attempts to improve conditions in the homes by development of cooperative arrangements between state hospitals and local adult homes, but it was not until 1978, with the introduction of the Community Support System (CSS) program that a formal program of state-funded, on-site services to the homes was developed.

The first program was a cooperative venture between the Bayview Manor Home (PPHA) and the South Beach Psychiatric Center (a New York State facility). South Beach developed an on-site team to work in the home providing care for the residents and working cooperatively with the management to improve conditions and the quality of life. This program was the first on-site rehabilitation program in New York State and served to provide psychiatric services and rehabilitation, to provide access to community-based mental health programs, and to link residents of the adult home to health care facilities and to various community activities. The relationship between the management of the home and the state team developed into a cooperative effort and included joint screening of new applicants. This cooperative relationship provided easy access to the South Beach Psychiatric Center for those adult home residents who needed rehospitalization, and generally improved the level of care in the facility. Creedmoor Psychiatric Center, another state facility in the New York City area, replicated this model and provided some on-site services to adult homes in Far Rockaway (Queens, New York City), where large numbers of former patients were housed.

In 1978 the establishment of the Community Support System by OMH provided an opportunity to develop large scale on-site rehabilitation programs. The plan enlisted the support of various private agencies, such as the Jewish Board of Family and Children's Services, Catholic Charities, Altro Workshops and the North Richmond Mental Health Centers, who would contractually provide needed health, mental health, and rehabilitation services, while simultaneously establishing on-site rehabilitation teams who would provide linkages to these services and to the nearest state psychiatric hospital. The adult home was now widely developed into a new institutional form that combined private ownership of the facility with publicly funded, voluntary agencies, and with state staff in on-site rehabilitation teams. An important element in the conceptual framework of the on-site teams was that by their presence they would affect continually the quality of life in the homes, as well as provide psychiatric, rehabilitation, and social services. The CSS program was made available not only to former patients who met the chronic patient criteria, but also to those who had functional disabilities and lived in a participating adult home, even though they had no qualifying psychiatric histories.

In discussions with adult home proprietors, management, and staff members and with on-site state team members, there has been support for the concept that heterogeneous groups of adult home residents can be managed, for the most part, with the collaborative arrangements of the management, the on-site teams, and the support of community agencies. A systematic evaluation of this program is currently in progress. However, anecdotal accounts of the experience are given below.

It was evident from talking with management, staff, and

on-site team members that their respective roles and the specific division of labor among them were not delineated. For example, while staff and team personnel cited poor personal hygiene of residents as a serious problem, and this was confirmed by assessment data (see Part II), it was not entirely clear who would assume responsibility for resident hygiene on a day-to-day basis. On-site teams of nurses, social workers, and psychologists, who were conducting activities of daily living training sessions, often were not specifically implementing these activities or supervising them. The implementation was not seen by them as part of their professional roles, and the staff of the home did not regard as it as their role either. In those few instances where on-site teams accepted such responsibility, they found this intervention to be a useful and effective means for changing resident behavior.

There seemed to be conflicting role perceptions in other areas as well. Staff of the homes sometimes perceived on-site team members as stressing verbal therapy and sometimes saw them as encouraging residents to become critical of conditions in the homes. Adult home staff also felt on-site teams should assume more responsibility for problems that arose with residents in relation to meals, housekeeping, and other routine activities. These were real obstacles to achieving treatment goals. However, while issues were present and unresolved, combined efforts of the team and the staff were effective and resulted in improved daily living activities, establishment of more formal programs, and escort services to community programs. These efforts ultimately resulted in lower community opposition to the homes and greater acceptance of mental patients.

Another area of great concern to the staff was how to keep the younger residents motivated to gain occupational skills when there were few jobs available and few sheltered workshop openings. Limitations on receiving additional income by SSI regulations also placed practical limits on the effectiveness of on-site programs and on maintaining and/or increasing resident motivation.

While the advantages of a heterogeneous population were noted, some problems were identified that resulted from the heterogeneity. For example, some younger residents had college educations and found routine and repetitious tasks boring. Some less vigorous residents found some activities of younger residents annoying. Team members cited problems with assaultive residents as being the most difficult, disruptive, and worrisome to staff and residents alike. They were quick to point out, however, that such assaultive behavior, while troublesome, was infrequent and usually manageable, and that, in many cases, the availability of on-site psychiatric consultation and crisis intervention served to diminish the need for some rehospitalizations.

This model appears to be viable and appropriate in addressing some previously unserved needs of residents of adult homes; however, it is only one type of possible intervention. There is an obvious need to develop and provide a broad and realistic range of opportunities and programs that will address the wide range of individual capacities and abilities represented by the residents of these homes. The important element here is the working partnership that was developed among the home proprietor, community agencies, and the state psychiatric facility, a relationship which improved quality of life for residents of adult homes.

The Case of the ICD Day Care Program

Kenneth Pommerenck, MASA

Cultural stereotypes tend to lump older people together and consider them very much alike. This is particularly true of the confused, disoriented older person with a diagnosis such as organic brain syndrome or senile dementia. In reality, each "senile" person is a unique human being waiting to be recognized and appreciated.

At the International Center for the Disabled there is a Day Center for older people who are suffering from confusion, disorientation, and memory loss: the so-called "senile" person and those who are dysfunctional as a result of situational factors. In operating this outpatient Day Center, techniques that had been developed and used successfully in inpatient settings are adapted for this special population. Persons who have given up, who have withdrawn, who have become desocialized, or who are acting out in various ways are encouraged to function as well as they possibly can in an accepting environment.

There are four full-time program staff and an average daily attendance of 20 participants. At any given time there are, in addition, approximately 15 volunteers assisting with the program. We also have a few visitors at any given time. The program is based on a therapeutic milieu. In structuring a therapeutic environment, everything in that environment is important. The space involved, the decor, layout, lighting, acoustics, and furnishings are all important, but the most important part of the environment is the people. Ask the people who are there. Each has an influence on the milieu and on the conduct of the others. That includes the clients and their personal relationships with each other. As they come to understand each other and respond to each other, they help each other and themselves.

In the ICD program there is an all-out effort to set up a positive attitude on the part of staff and volunteers toward the participants in the program. This in turn acts to bring about a positive attitude in the participants toward staff and volunteers. Many participants are extremely anxious when they come into the program. They are almost completely dependent on a family caretaker, and some cannot be out of sight of their relative without becoming agitated. The intake is relaxed and informal. A casual exploratory visit to the program is encouraged. Participants are treated as welcome guests.

All of the activities in the program are part of an environment that is highly structured and has as an important objective facilitating day-to-day functions. Meal planning, shopping, and meal preparation are integral and very essential parts of the program. Activities such as memory games, word games, and pricing games are hard work. Each day begins with a discussion of what has occurred since the last session at the Center, and each day ends with a discussion regarding what has gone on that day.

Two important techniques in the Day Center milieu are Reality Orientation and Attitude Therapy. Reality Orientation is a rehabilitation approach in which the environment is structured to reinforce continually facts of time, place, and person and to encourage self-activation and decision making. Developed under the leadership of Dr. James C. Folsom, it began as a search for a therapeutic role for aides and attendants in mental institutions and is enjoying continued evolution and broader application.

Reality Orientation has not been well understood. Too many people see it as a simplistic, mechanical process wherein a group of "senile" people takes turns reading a reality board, i.e., a board containing basic orientation information such as time and place. In fact, it is not the information itself but rather the quality of the personal relationship that is important. Furthermore, it is necessary that Reality Orientation be applied and reinforced 24 hours a day by everyone coming in contact with the impaired person.

Attitude Therapy originated at the Menninger Foundation. It is based on the concept that the manner in which things are said and the atmosphere created through our actions may be even more important than what we say. There are five attitudes which are prescribed by the treatment team to meet the needs of the individual.

Attitude Therapy is a form of behavioral modification that is usually used in conjunction with Reality Orientation. This form of therapy is designed to establish definite attitudes in working with five established behavior patterns of elderly patients. The goals are to reinforce desirable behavior and eliminate undesirable behavior.

The five major attitudes are:

1. *Kind firmness* is prescribed for depressive elderly patients. These patients have turned their anger inward. They are assigned menial tasks, and these tasks are in turn criticized by the staff. Sympathy is not offered to the patients' feeling of worthlessness or despair.
2. *Active friendliness* is used with individuals who are withdrawn and apathetic. Attention is given to the patient before he requests it. Failure from accomplishments is prevented as much as possible. This attitude is most typically prescribed for patients in Reality Orientation.
3. *Passive friendliness* is prescribed for those who are distrustful and frightened by closeness and/or active friendliness. Staff wait for the patient to make the first move and then respond accordingly.
4. *No demand* is designed to work with patients who are suspicious, frightened, or in an uncontrollable rage. Staff expectation of patients' safety is exhibited as a priority.
5. *Matter-of-fact* is used to work with manipulative and seductive patients, as well as for those approaching normal behavior. Responses to patient behavior are consistent, casual, and calm. (Barnes et al., 1973)

In working with the confused and disoriented person, it enables staff to simplify the environment greatly by feeding back the same attitude and consistent responses to the patient. This replaces the confusing messages most patients struggle with as different staff present their individual and conflicting ideas of what the person can or cannot do and should or should not do. Consistency avoids nontherapeutic interventions, such as the patient who is strongly urged to walk on one shift and persuaded to stay in a wheelchair on another shift or the patient who is fed on one shift and eats by himself on another. The ability to adapt to different staff expectations is rarely seen by staff as a strength on which to build. In fact, without the team approach to care, it may not even be noticed.

This positive, expectant approach is reality based. It does not deny or ignore whatever irreversible condition may be present. Rather, it asserts the fact that the observed dysfunction has a variety of causes. These include fear, anxiety, frustration, and learned helplessness. Of course, individual differences must be taken into account at all times.

If there is something in the course of the day's activities which triggers in a participant an unusual behavior, it is dealt with. For example:

> In a loud tone of voice one program participant suddenly demanded to be taken home, "I have to go home. My mother is sick. She is there and she needs me." I asked the lady if we could talk about it. I told her this was puzzling since she had told me before that she left Hungary as a young girl and left her parents and brothers and sisters behind. She nodded and said that I was right. We talked a bit more and she suddenly said, "I have to go home because my father is there and he needs me." Again, we explored whether or not her father actually was there or could be there. Instead of acknowledging directly that he was not, she said her son was home from school and she had to go. I responded that a few months ago she had become a grandmother for the second time, that her son is married and he and his wife now have two children. At this point she started to cry softly, and she said, "Sometimes I don't know what world I'm living in."

If we can help to make the present tolerable, there is much less need for the patient/client to regress. Taking control of one's life again and making responsible decisions are acts that we strongly encourage.

One man had severe problems before entering the program. He became lost going to his daughter's apartment the day they were to come for intake. He was very disorganized and constantly misplacing his newspaper, his hat, and his jacket. His life was in shambles.

We worked together to find organizational systems he could use. He got a pocket calendar and learned to keep it. He used a system of clip boards at home to keep things in some order. He received counselling to help him work through the death of his wife a few months before and the trauma of giving up their home and taking a small apartment. His daughter helped him to get an efficiency apartment in a senior citizens housing complex. He told us what he needed to have help with.

One day about 5 months after he entered the program, he said, "Ken, when do you people realize when someone doesn't need you any more?" I replied, "I guess when they tell us. Are you telling us?"

He met a retired nurse and they fell in love. Their plans for marriage were interrupted when he suffered a fatal stroke, but he died happy and free and oriented to the future.

Very few of our participants experience dramatic improvements due to the nature of the underlying disease process; however, the program does seem to improve the quality of life for an often overburdened family and for a patient who has become desocialized, at the least, if not totally isolated.

Mobilizing the Family

Miriam K. Aronson, EdD

There is not only a graying of the American population in general but also a dramatic decrease in the mortality rate of the very old. In the past 10 years, the mortality of those over 80 has declined by an impressive 25% (Rosenwaike, 1980). Thus more people are living into old age to begin with, and the very old are living longer than ever before. If this trend continues, there will be an ever-growing number of very old persons. Considering that those persons over the age of 75 are increasingly at risk for the ravages of disease, this trend has tremendous social and also economic implications.

Little attention is paid to the quality of life of older persons in our society. For example, there is poor housing at the outset, and this certainly interferes with function and adaptation, and ultimately with health and well-being. There are disparate sources of funding for similar services and sometimes no funding at all for needed services. Furthermore, uneven and/or unrealistic eligibility criteria or restrictions contribute to chaotic service utilization patterns. As a matter of fact, some say that there really is no system. Rather, there are parallel systems, i.e., the health care delivery system, the social service delivery system, and the family. These systems of care all coexist and sometimes compete for clients and for funds. While the clients may be similar, each system has its own bias, and, as a result, persons of similar need may receive entirely different services. For example, a moderately demented older person may be in a skilled nursing facility or maintained at home by family with no outside services or funding.

The "system" of health care delivery itself is quite imperfect. There are several barriers to health care for older persons. There are financial barriers which have not been solved by Medicare. There are geographical barriers which have increased with the increasing tendency toward specialization and centralization. The system is fraught with unclear entry points which serve to limit access. Moreover, there appears to be insensitivity of those who work in the system to the special needs of the older persons they are supposed to be serving. In the long-term care system, there is a bias toward institutional care, and most resources are concentrated on nursing home care, despite the fact that there are many elderly in the community with heavy care needs. In fact, for every person in a nursing home, there are at least another 2.5 persons of a similar impairment level living in the community.

The social service system is also fraught with difficulties. Access points are often unclear. Eligibility requirements may vary from program to program and place to place. Medicaid is a classic example, for requirements vary from state to state. Also, separate applications may be necessary for specific benefit programs, e.g., food stamps, rent subsidies. It is often logistically difficult for a frail person to obtain his/her benefit entitlements since he/she may be required to make multiple trips to bureaucratic offices in a variety of locations. It is not surprising, therefore, that family members usually serve as outreach agents and mediators of the bureaucratic system (Sussman, 1976; Dunlop, 1980).

Contrary to the prevailing myths regarding vanishing families and abandoned old persons, various surveys (Shanas et al., 1968; Cantor, 1976) have revealed that at the least, there is usually a family member who lives less than one hour away who is available not only to mediate the system, but also as a first line of defense in times of crisis. Families do not usually contact the formal system until they have exhausted their own means of resolution of crisis. Thus, despite the existence of a large and costly formal service system, there is an even larger, pervasive yet often unrecognized functional system of informal supports (Sussman, 1976). It is these informal supports which prevent the long-term care system from becoming bankrupt.

Though these mutual aid arrangements may appear to be idyllic, they are not without problems. There often are tugs between and among at least three generations, with the middle group (the adult children) feeling the pinch. These adult children may themselves be aging and might be experiencing physical decrements associated with aging and illness while they struggle to assist their teenage children and simultaneously to tend to the needs of their aged parents. Elderly spouses may simply be physically incapable of assuming total care for their impaired counterpart even though they really want to. Caretakers may be overworked and overwhelmed in the face of unrelenting needs for care of a loved one. There is, in fact, reported to be a higher than normal incidence of depression and other stress-related illness among caretakers. How long does an overstressed family try to keep a relative out of an institution?

Not only are there considerable physical demands on caretaking relatives, there are considerable emotional costs. As in all chronic illnesses, there are a range of reactions and issues that arise among them, i.e., denial, anger, ambivalence, and guilt. Issues of dependency and role reversals may exacerbate long-standing unresolved conflicts in relationships. Behaviors may be affected by these feelings and may deteriorate. As a result, while enlisting the aid of the kinship network, the formal system may have to aid simultaneously those family members who are beset with problems themselves while trying to provide ongoing care and support.

Placement is not a quick answer for these emotional woes. In fact, it comes with a myriad of problems. Because of the lack of clarity of the placement process, myriad issues around placement, and the lack of available emotional support for families, families may become estranged from their institutionalized acting-out relatives. Often it is this estrangement and the consequent lack of social supports which perpetuate the need for continued institutionalization—thus creating a vicious cycle which feeds on itself. Institutionalization does not obviate the need for families. In fact, mental hospital staff query: How do you reinvolve an estranged family after many years of noninvolvement? Nursing home staff ask: How do you keep the level of interest up in relatives of a nursing home population so that they come to visit regularly? Adult home operators ask: How do you maintain better cooperation between family and adult home residents?

How then do you mobilize families? There is no simple answer; however, there are a variety of strategies that may be useful.

Potentially Useful Strategies for Working with Families

Categorical disease self-help groups have been helpful to family members of all ages. There are many such groups organizing in various communities, around various problems—Alcoholics Anonymous and Alzheimer's Disease and Related Disorders Association. These groups serve to educate people about the disease process, to provide a forum for ventilation of angry feelings, and to provide a basis for mutual support among peers. These groups are usually run by family members, with or without professional consultation.

Special short-term groups, e.g., groups for families of newly admitted nursing home residents, groups for families of newly diagnosed cancer patients, may be of similar value. These are usually professionally led, short term, and goal oriented and may be offered in conjunction with services for the afflicted person.

Family therapy and/or counselling may be indicated where unresolved feelings and conflicts are interfering with appropriate treatment or management of family members. Family meetings with professionals may help to gather the strength to implement needed interventions for frail older persons.

Family role maintenance must be accomplished. Support the family to maintain its ties by participating in various aspects of patient care. At home, the spouse usually supervises the surrogate caretaker and is able to maintain a sense of purpose, in the presence of assistance with the actual physical tasks involved in care. When the loved one is placed in an institutional facility, even though the physical care has now been relegated to the institutional staff, the spouse needs to provide continued emotional support, love, and affection for the partner. Visiting should be encouraged, as well as participation in various aspects of care.

Families may be encouraged to sponsor various activities such as birthday and holiday parties, to assist with feedings, and to support other patients who have no families.

Respite services are extremely valuable—*relief* for the overstressed person for rest or recreation—be it for a few hours, a few days, or even a few weeks once in a while. These may consist of in-home services by a temporary caregiver-surrogate or may be temporary residential placement for the afflicted person at a community facility. Currently, these services are available either on a demonstration grant basis or on a private basis, where families make their own financial arrangements. No third-party reimbursement is available at this time, though it is sorely needed.

Home care services by housekeepers and/or home attendants may enable the family to assume the responsibility for care for a longer period of time before placement in an institution becomes necessary. Encouragement of the family to accept help of this nature, if only on a limited basis, may be an important aspect of therapeutic intervention.

Financial incentives are not available at this time to encourage family care. As a matter of fact, there are probably more disincentives at this time than incentives.

Changes in public policy are necessary to acknowledge and encourage the role of families in the provision of services for the elderly. Intervention to support these family activities could conceivably be more cost-effective than trying to build more institutions.

In summary, I do not believe that families do not want to take care of their elderly. Many do—and work very hard at it. In fact, in my practice, I see firsthand the devastation that can be wrought on a family by a long-term, progressive, debilitating disease, such as Alzheimer's disease. I also see the dilemmas that our public policy poses with its institutional bias.

There are no quick answers. That is a problem; but maybe therein lies the solution: What is desperately needed is mobilization of a supportive working relationship between and among the health care system, the social service system, and the family.

Part VI

SUMMARY AND CONCLUSIONS

Summary and Conclusions

Miriam K. Aronson, EdD
Ruth Bennett, PhD
Barry J. Gurland, MD, MRCP

In trying to summarize, one thing is abundantly clear: The "acting-out" elderly are not a single entity but rather a heterogeneous group of individuals within a heterogeneous group of individuals we have come to call the frail elderly. These are not typical older persons but rather many types of deviant older persons with special problems and special needs.

All of us are involved with this group, whether as lay persons or as professionals. Whether we encounter the bag lady or the elderly alcoholic on the street corner, in the supermarket, or in the subway or whether they are served by us through our institutions or agencies, they are part of our lives.

This is a group of people who is generally rejected by their peers and occasionally may be dangerous to themselves or others. This is a group that frustrates helping professionals of all disciplines. This is a group that is often estranged from their families. This is a group that may at times challenge not only the patience of those working in the system but the system itself.

From our brief exploration of service models which are used to deal with the acting-out elderly, it is apparent that we play it by ear, dealing almost on a case-by-case basis, picking and choosing who is to be served. Currently, various modalities are utilized—the family, traditional social and health agencies, and innovative programs such as those described here, i.e., mobile crisis teams, community support teams, and day care programs. It becomes abundantly clear that highly specialized programs targeted toward acting-out behavior are not well developed as yet, and it is recommended that research efforts be geared toward developing systematic approaches to acting-out behaviors in the elderly. Given the demographic trends of increased survival by older persons despite the ravages of age and chronic disease, it would appear that the number of persons of this type will increase. Given the current climate of deinstitutionalization and the generally increased competition for fewer services due to limitations in funding, it is likely that their needs will remain largely unmet in the coming years. Though their needs have not yet been delineated, it appears that they are multidimensional and largely unmet. Their situation is by no means static; nor are their needs. Because of the complexity and the unpredictability of their situations, there cannot be one single agency or even one single strategy to deal with this group. What is needed instead is a broad-based, multifaceted flexible approach. Following are recommendations for action.

Clearly, there must be *recognition* of the fact that the frail elderly are a heterogeneous group with a diversity of problems and needs. There is need to identify the nature and scope of the problems. It must also be recognized that the subgroup of frail elderly whom we have labeled the "hard-to-manage" or "acting-out" may have distinct perceptions of their needs, and these perceptions may differ markedly from those of the persons who are trying to provide services for this group.

Secondly, there is need for some *epidemiological information*. Since many of them are not involved with the service system or with the typical statistics, gathering agencies many undoubtedly escape notice. This group must be better defined. Subgroups such as alcoholics and street people have been mentioned here but not discussed in depth. Third, there is also need for delineation of the legal and ethical considerations that may be involved in serving an unwilling or an otherwise difficult population. It would appear that new services and programs may not be the answer. Rather there is need for greater flexibility within existing programs to accommodate varying needs. Special services such as protective services must be better defined.

Fourth, a massive educational effort is needed. Information about this group must be included in a variety of curricula and in both formal and informal training modalities in gerontology and in long-term care. At minimum, the following should be included:

1. Information regarding the type and prevalence of the problems of the frail elderly.
2. Information regarding strategies for assessment. Very often the real problems are masked and therefore missed. For example, there is a need to separate those with long-standing problems from those with recent difficulties, those with irrevocable causes as compared with those with remediable ones.
3. Training regarding strategies for crisis intervention. While this may not be the orthodox or comprehensive approach, it may often be the most pragmatic and perhaps a needed first step to increased intervention.
4. Training in multidisciplinary/interdisciplinary practice. Since the problems cross disciplinary lines, it is usually necessary for cooperative interventions by various helping professionals/paraprofessionals.
5. Training about deviance—alcoholism, drug dependency, suicide, mental illness, and retardation.
6. Training about dementing illness.
7. Training for information, referral, and advocacy work.

Fifth, this group would benefit greatly from our constructing and/or rebuilding informal supports. Current social policies tend to discourage family involvement. We would like to see this reversed. Specifically, we would like to see psychological support services for caretaking families as well as tax incentives, if not direct stipends, for family caregivers.

Further, while professionals and/or paraprofessionals from a multiplicity of disciplines may be interested in this group, interdisciplinary involvement is needed. We need not only the traditional health and social service professionals but also lawyers and ethicists, pharmacists, housing officials, clergy, and economists, to name some of the key groups.

Moreover, we need desperately to come to some resolution regarding the issue of forcing services. There are ethical questions involved: patients rights, informed consent, the right to refuse treatment, society's rights. We need to look at our current Protective Services System. These services are protective for whom and for what? Moreover, whatever they are, they are in very short supply. How should they be expanded? How could they be simplified? For example, how could competency proceedings be streamlined? Here we could also use input from legislators and judges.

In these times of shrinking services all of these strategies may become even more important in that there will be a shrinking group of providers for a growing group of needy individuals. Where to start? Perhaps conferences such as this one are a most sensible first step.

Bibliography

Atchley, R. Aging and suicide: Reflection of the quality of life? In S. Haynes and M. Feinleib (eds.), *Proceedings of the Second Conference on the Epidemiology of Aging.* Washington, DC: U.S. Government Printing Office, 1980.

Atkinson, J. The Samaritans and the elderly. In *Proceedings of the 5th International Congress of Suicide Prevention.* London, 1970.

Bagley, C. The evaluation of a suicide prevention scheme by an ecological method. *Soc. Sci. Med.*, 1968, *2*, 1–14.

Bagley, C. Authoritarianism, status integration and suicide. *Sociology*, 1972, *6*, 395–404.

Bagley, C. Suicide prevention by the Samaritans. *Lancet*, 1977, *2*, 348–349.

Barns, E. K., Sack, A., and Shore, H. Guidelines to treatment approaches: Modalities and methods for use with the aged. *The Gerontologist*, 1973, *13*(4), 513–527.

Barraclough, B. Suicide in the elderly. In D. Kay and A. Walk (eds.), *Recent developments in psychogeriatrics.* London: Royal Medico-Psychological Association, 1971.

Barraclough, B. Suicide prevention, recurrent affective disorder and lithium. *Brit. J. Psychiat.*, 1972, *121*, 391–392.

Barraclough, B., Bunch J., Nelson, B., and Sainsbury, P. A hundred cases of suicide: Clinical aspects. *Brit. J. Psychiat.*, 1974, *125*, 355–373.

Barraclough, B., and Pallis, D. Depression followed by suicide: A comparison of depressed suicides with living depressives. *Psychological Medicine*, 1975, *5*, 55–61.

Baxter, E., and Hopper, K. *Private lives/public spaces, homeless adults on the streets of New York City.* New York: Community Services, Society, 1981.

Bennett, R. (Ed.). *Aging, isolation and resocialization.* New York: Van Nostrand Reinhold, 1980.

Bennett, R., and Cook, D. Social isolation of the aged in New York City, in planning for the elderly in N.Y.C., *Proceedings of a Research Utilization Workshop.* New York: Community Council of Greater New York, 1980.

Berkman, B. Community mental health services for the elderly. *Community Mental Health Review*, 1977, *2*(3).

Blank, M. L. A perspective on de-institutionalization of older persons and a proposal for community-based services. *Journal of Gerontological Social Work*, 1978, *1*(2), 135–145.

Bridge, T., Potkin, S., Zung, W. et al. Suicide prevention centers: Ecological study of effectiveness. *J. Nerv. Ment. Dis.*, 1977, *164*, 18–24.

Brody, E. Serving the aged: Educational needs as viewed by practice. *Social Work*, October 1970.

Brown, J. Suicide in Britain, more attempts, fewer deaths, lessons for public policy. *Arch. Gen. Psychiat.*, 1979, *36*, 1119–1124.

Bultena, G., and Powers, E. A. Denial of aging: Age identification and reference group orientation. *J. of Gerontology*, 1970, *34*(3), 423–428.

Burr, H. T. Working with mentally impaired center members. In *Working with the impaired elderly*. The National Council on Aging, 1976.

Butler, R. N., and Lewis, M. I. *Aging and mental health*. St. Louis: C. V. Mosby, 1977.

Cameron, P. Suicide and the generation gap. *Life-threatening Behavior*, 1972, *2*, 194–208.

Cantor, M., and Mayer, M. Health and the inner city elderly. *Gerontologist*, 1976, *16*(1), 17–25.

Comfort, A. *A good age*. New York: Crown Publications, 1976.

Dobrof, R., and Litwak, E. *Maintenance of family ties of long term care patients*. Rockville, MD: U.S. Dept. of Health and Human Services, 1981.

Dunlop, B. D. Expanded home-based care for the frail elderly: Solution or pipe-dream. *American Journal of Public Health*, 1980, *70*(5), 514–519.

Durkheim, E. (1897) *Suicide*. J. Spaulding, G. Simpson (trans.) Glencoe, IL: Free Press, 1951.

Erikson, E. *Childhood and society*. New York: W. W. Norton, 1950.

Farberow, N., and McEvoy, E. Suicide among patients with diagnosis of anxiety reaction or depressive reaction in general medical and surgical hospitals. *J. Abnormal and Social Psychology*, 1966, *71*, 287–299.

Farberow, N., and Shneidman, E. Suicide and age. In E. Shneidman and N. Farberow (eds.), *Clues to suicide*. New York: McGraw-Hill, 1957.

Federal Council on Aging. *Public policy and the frail elderly*. Washington, DC: U.S. Dept. of HEW, 1978.

Federal Council on the Aging. *Mental health and the elderly: Recommendations for action*. Washington, DC: U.S. Dept. of HEW, 1979.

Fogel, R. W., Hatfield, E., Kiesler, S. B., and Shanas, E. (eds). *Aging: Stability and change in the family*. New York: Academic Press, 1981.

Gardner, E., Bahn, A., and Mack, M. Suicide and psychiatric care in the aging. *Arch. Gen. Psychiat.*, 1964, *10*, 546–553.

Golden, Sister J. *Discovering th hidden elderly in the invisible elderly*. Washington, DC: National Council on the Aging, Inc., 1976.

Gruenberg, E. N., Snow, H. B., and Bennett, C. L. Preventing the social breakdown syndrome. In F. C. Redeich (ed.), *Social psychiatry*. Baltimore: Williams and Wilkins Co., 1969.

Gurland, B., and Cross, P. The epidemiology of psychopathology in old age. Some implications for clinical services. *Psychiatric Clinics of North America*, 1982, *5*(1).

Gurland, B., Copeland, J., Kuriansky, J., Kelleher, M., Sharpe, E., and Dean, L. *The mind and mood of aging*. New York: Haworth Press, in press.

Gurland, B., and Toner, J. Depression in the elderly: A 1981 review. In *Annual review of gerontology and geriatrics*, Vol. 3, 1981.

Harris, C. S. *Fact book on aging: A profile of America's older population*. Washington, DC: National Council on the Aging, Inc., 1978.

Hinsie, L. E., and Campbell, R. J. *Psychiatric dictionary*. New York: Oxford University Press, 1960.
Jacobs, B. *Senior centers and the at-risk older person*. Washington, DC: National Council on the Aging, Inc., 1980.
Jupa, R. Bronx Mobile Geriatrics Crisis Intervention Unit, Report on Second Year, April 1, 1977 – March 31, 1978.
Katzman, R., and Karasu, T. B. Differential diagnosis of dementia. In W. Fields (ed.), *Neurological and sensory disorders of the elderly*. Miami, FL: Symposia Specialists, 1975.
Kobrynski, B. The mentally impaired elderly—Whose responsibility? *Gerontologist*, October 1975.
Kohut, H. *The restoration of the self*. New York: International Universities Press, Inc., 1977.
Lawton, M. P. *Social and medical services in housing for the aged*. Rockville, MD: Department of Health and Human Services, 1980.
Low, A., Farmer, R., Jones, D., and Rohde, J. Suicide in England and Wales: An analysis of 100 years, 1876–1975. *Psychological Medicine*, 1981, *11*, 359–368.
Lester, D. Effects of suicide prevention centers on suicide rates in the United States. *Health Service Rep.*, 1974, *89*, 37–39.
Maletta, G. et al. Organic mental disorders in a geriatric outpatient. *American Journal of Psychiatry*, 1982, *4*, 521.
Marshall, J. Changes in the aged white male suicide: 1948–1972. *J. Geront.*, 1978, *33*, 763–768.
Mirotznick, J. S. A sociological analysis of a relocation process. Unpublished PhD dissertation, Rutgers, the State University of New Jersey, 1978.
Mishara, B. L., and Kastenbaum, R. *Alcohol and old age*. New York: Grune and Stratton, 1980.
Moryez, R. K. An exploration of senile dementia and family burden. *Clinical Social Work Journal*, 1980, *8*(1).
Murphy, G. The physician's responsibility for suicide: 1. An error of commission and 2. Errors of omission. *Ann. Intern. Med.*, 1975, *82*, 301–309.
Nelson, F., and Farberow, N. Indirect suicide in the elderly chronically ill patient. In K. Achte and J. Lonngvist (eds.), *Suicide research*. Helsinki: Psychiatria Fennica, 1977.
Nelson, F., and Farberow, N. Indirect self-destructive behavior in the elderly nursing home patient. *J. Geront.*, 1980, *35*, 949–959.
New York Mental Hygiene Law. Secs. 9.01, 9.27, 9.39, McKinney's Consolidated Laws of New York, Book 34A. St. Paul: West Publishing Co., 1978.
Protective Services for Adults, Bulletin #194. New York: New York State Department of Social Services, 1982.
Robins, E., Murphy G., Wilkinson, R., Glassner, S., and Kayes, J. Some clinical considerations in the prevention of suicide based on a study of 134 successful suicides. *Amer. J. Pub. Health*, 1959, *49*, 888–898.
Rodstein, M., Savitsky, E., and Starkman, R. Initial adjustment to a long

term care institution: Behavioral aspects. *J. Am. Geriat. Soc.*, 1976, *24*(12), 65–71.

Rosenwaike, I., Yaffe, N., and Sagi, P. C. The recent decline in mortality of the extreme aged: An analysis of statistical data. *American Journal of Public Health*, 1980, *70*(10), 1074–1080.

Sainsbury, P. *Suicide in London.* London: Chapman and Hall, 1955.

Sainsbury, P. Social and epidemiological aspects of suicide with special reference to the aged. In R. Williams, C. Tibbitts, and W. Donahue (eds.), *Processes of aging, II.* New York: Atherton Press, 1963.

Sainsbury, P. Suicide and depression. In A. Coppen and A. Walk (eds.), *Recent developments in affective disorders. Brit. J. Psychiat.*, special publication no. 2, 1968.

Shanas, E., Townsend, D., Wedderburn, D., Friis, H., Milhoj, P., and Stehouwer, J. *Old people in three industrial societies.* New York: Atherton Press, 1968.

Soyer, David. The geriatric patient and his family: Helping the family to live with itself. *Journal of Geriatric Psychiatry*, 1972, *5*(1).

Sussman, M. B. The family life of old people. In R. H. Binstock and E. Shanas (eds.), *Handbook of aging and the social sciences.* New York: Van Nostrand Reinhold, 1976.

Turner, B. F., Tobin, S. S., and Lieberman, M. A. Personality traits as predictors of institutional adaptation among the aged. *Journal of Gerontology*, 1972, *27*(1), 61–68.

Vladeck, B. *Unloving care: The nursing home tragedy.* New York: Basic Books, 1980.

Walk, D. Suicide and community care. *Brit. J. Psychiat.*, 1967, *113*, 1381–1391.

Welu, T. A follow-up program for suicide attempters: Evaluation of effectiveness. *Suicide and Life-Threatening Behavior*, 1977, 7, 17–30.

Wilder, D. The assessment of chronically depressed—Results of a longitudinal study. In *Planning for the elderly in New York City.* New York: Community Council of Greater New York, 1980.

Winokur, G., and Tsuang, M. The Iowa 500: Suicide in mania, depression, and schizophrenia. *Amer. J. Psychiat.*, 1975, *132*, 650–651.